What people are saying about Food Fix:

"In an enjoyable, easy-to-read format, Susan Lebel Young offers a lifesaving book for people who suffer from 'food frenzy.' Through the lens of counselor, mindfulness coach, and fellow traveler, she connects with the confusion and fear of those imprisoned by food. Food frenzy is a difficult, multi-dimensional issue, and Susan Young tackles it with several approaches, including nutrition that heals, suggested practices for developing 'heartfulness,' and a journal-like approach that depicts the author's struggle at various life stages. Quotes scattered throughout the text and the bibliography are delightful bonuses."

> —Joanne Turnbull, PhD, Founding Partner, Your Write Mind and Executive Director, Emerita National Patient Safety Foundation

"*Food Fix* will help you get underneath food cravings, habits, and old behaviors that are holding you back and keeping you from being as vibrant and radiant as you would like. Susan speaks with deep experience, passion, and great care about what total health means: body, mind and heart. Page by page, chapter by chapter, she teaches the miracles of self-nourishment. This is extraordinarily helpful in this food-crazed culture. And for an added side-effect...this way of living and eating can also improve our global health crisis."

> —Julieanna Hever, MS, RD, CPT, www.PlantBasedDietitian.com

"Savor this book. Take your time with it. It's the real thing, filled with the kind of wisdom that only comes from the trenches. Sue Young brings a depth of understanding to the complex food issues that entrap and entangle so many of us today. After her wholehearted efforts, over the course of decades, she has emerged from the maze and the fog to offer guidance for others who are struggling with the food koan. Sue's voice is clear, strong and beautiful and her message is grounded in wisdom. I love this book."

> —Linda Anderson Krech, LICSW, ToDo Institute

"*Food Fix* offers an amazingly corrective, functional and heartfelt approach to food, eating and self-care."   —Joseph McLeod, BA, CPT, FMS

"This is a courageous book. By sharing her personal journey, Susan inspires hope for a gentle, self-compassionate way out of what she calls 'Food Frenzy'. With each chapter's Antidotes to Food Frenzy, she is right there with her reader, teaching and encouraging from beginning to end of this valuable book. (I've already established a new morning ritual, based on what I learned in Chapter Twelve.) *Food Fix* shows us the importance and healing power of mindfulness."

—Maggie Butler, MSW Writer and Co-Founder, Your Write Mind, P.A.
www.yourwritemind.net

"If you are ready to break free from the seduction of unhealthful foods, this is the book for you. Susan Young shares valuable lessons from her journey to overcome dependence on high-fat, sugary foods and gives you the tools you need to take control of your health. Refocusing your menu on healthful fruits, vegetables, whole grains, and legumes will change your life. Susan will inspire you to nourish yourself."

—Neal Barnard, President, Physicians Committee for Responsible Medicine

"This is a wonderful book. *Food Fix* is not another diet book. Rather it is a "life" book. It points to the only place you can really find nourishment and contentment which is in your heart. It's fair to say - food is important, the body needs it to live, but it can never fulfill the longing to be whole and healed. That comes from within you. This is a work of a lifetime, may you fare well in the journey."

—Bob Stahl, Ph.D. co-author of *A Mindfulness-Based Stress Reduction Workbook, Living With Your Heart Wide Open,* and *Calming the Rush of Panic*

"*Food Fix* fills a gap in the resources available to individuals interested in healing their relationship to food. The emphasis on Heartfulness provides a grounding center of kindness and compassion in the process of "getting real with food." Sue befriends the reader by sharing her personal experiences, peppered with cultural references to create a bridge of trust through shared humanity. She takes the reader by the hand and—one chapter at a time—builds a pathway toward self-awareness and access to inner knowing. The blend of ancient teachings and action steps empower the readers to discern real nourishment and find their way home to themselves."

—Julie Gray, R.N.

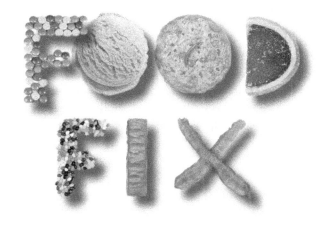

Ancient Nourishment
For Modern Hungers

SUSAN LEBEL YOUNG

MSED MSC

FOREWORD BY JOHN ROBBINS

A desperate search for answers limits your perspective. Next time, why don't you stop searching and just have a heartful conversation with your question.

—Rainer Maria Rilke

Library of Congress Catalog Card No.: 2012948941

Young, Susan Lebel
Food Fix: Ancient Nourishment for Modern Hungers

Susan Lebel Young
p. 204
1. Health & Fitness : Healthy Living. 2. Self-Help : Personal Growth - Success.
3. Body, Mind & Spirit : Inspiration & Personal Growth
I. Title.

Softcover: 978-1-934949-52-8
ebook: 978-1-934949-65-8

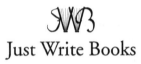

Just Write Books
www.jstwrite.com
Topsham, ME 04086
Printed in the United States of America

Dedication

Food Fix is dedicated to the millions of us caught, over and over again, in newfangled modern diet ideas. This book is also dedicated to those in doubt about what, when, why or where to eat, and to those desperately searching for a heartful conversation about the huge suffering caused by those confusing questions.

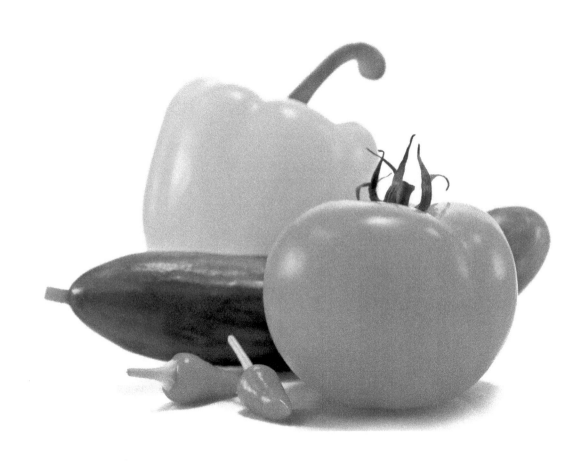

Contents

Part One
Awakening and Getting Real

Part Two
Returning Home Again and Again

Part Three
Staying Awake

Part Four
Silence

Acknowledgements

And now here is my secret, a very simple secret: it is only with the
heart that one can see rightly; what is essential is invisible to the eye.
—Antoine de Saint-Exupéry

On the one hand, I did not make up heartfulness; not the word, not the concepts,
not the practices. I learned it through years of working with gifted mindfulness
teachers who stressed compassion. Many of them are listed in the bibliography.

On the other hand, I made up how the work of the heart healed my food
frenzy. Like ingredients in a stew that no longer can be seen as individual parts,
my work became a larger-than-life recipe, or maybe more like a cookbook, or even
maybe more like how to live in a new home. In that sense, I take full responsibility
for any mis-use or misinterpretation of the ancient sacred heart-opening ways of
being. Any mistaken ideas about them are mine. This is my story, embedded in a
large cultural story of trouble with how to fully nourish ourselves. I hope how I
cooked up the ingredients for me helps you savor your life too.

I am deeply grateful to those whose work and whose whole being have
taught me to see with the heart:

My family: My daughter Alisa with husband Coley and children, Walker,
Taylor and Lawson Andrews, who are creating the most heartful family I know;
my son, Zac Young who has always followed his heart and Jon Young, my
spouse, who fills my heart in every moment.

The men and women of the on-going Tuesday night group, who for five
years studied yoga, mindfulness and meditation with me. For your open hearts,
bright minds and beautiful spirits, thank you.

The Friday morning group, Maureen McQuade, Joan Perkins, Carroll

Acknowledgements

Tiernan, Carol Goloff, Cheryl Cameron: Thank you for your brilliance and patience as you helped me go through chapter after chapter of this book, finding typos and inconsistencies and challenging me to write in closer to what I really mean.

Sunday writing group. I so appreciate Joan Hunter for developing in me the heart of a writer. And many big hugs to Nancy Coleman, Susan Gassett, Deb Harlow, Corinne Martin, Marcel Moreau and Dulcie Witman, my fellow Sunday writers, for careful reading and firm yet gentle critiquing of early drafts of the manuscript.

Richard and Diane Herman for deep and long friendship and for countless nights of listening to me talk on and on about this project.

My teachers at the Center for Mindfulness: Jon Kabat-Zinn PhD, who introduced me to the word "heartfulness" and whose writings and teachings began this journey for me and for millions across the world.

Saki Santorelli, EDd, whose first assignment to us in the Center for Mindfulness' first ever Teacher Development Intensive was "Begin to notice the openings and closings of your heart."

Ferris Urbanowski MFA, whose main message to me when she noticed how hard and harsh I could be toward myself was, " Mercy, mercy, mercy."

Nancy Carlson, PhD, who was the first to say, "Move the energy to your heart."

Jack McCall, Episcopal priest and Zen monk who was the first to tell me I think too much.

Bob Stahl, PhD, who re-iterated: "no mind, no problem."

T. Colin Campbell and Cornell for three on-line plant-based nutrition courses and on-going work that transformed my relationship to food.

John Robbins, for mentoring, for role-modeling, for just the right words in his beautiful foreword.

Howard Lyman, Caldwell and Rip Esselstyn, men of great intellect, integrity and compassion, who followed the heart of the science and dared to speak the

Acknowledgements

plant-based truth, facing the danger of losing careers and family.

Julie Gray for always reminding me to soften, to invite tenderness and who offers me the deepest teachings I know.

Joe McLeod, personal trainer, for honoring my body as it shows up in present moment time, two days a week for years now, through injuries and through my grandiose ideas of just how hard to train.

Julieanna Hever, plant-based dietician extraordinaire who wrote a leafy-green blurb for the book, and who keeps reminding me about creating the best of health, "You can do this. It's easier than you're making this. When you get hungry, eat a whole plant food. If you're not hungry enough to eat an apple, you're probably not really hungry."

Dean Ornish for his work in opening the heart in both physical and metaphoric ways, for teaching us all that what we feed ourselves matters on all levels.

Teena Zimmerman, PhD, for being my friend, for listening, for telling the truth.

Tanja Kunz for her whole-foods, low-fat, plant-based teaching, her inspiration, and her role modeling.

Gregg Krech and Linda Anderson Krech of the ToDo Institute, for teaching us all about the power of gratitude, simplicity, self-reflection and living life with purpose. Their reminder to "do what needs doing" helped me take one step after another for this project.

Marcia G. Hutchinson, now a web magician, who years ago gave me my first mantra: "This is my body. This is where I live."

Nancy E. Randolph, publisher and friend, for her time and talent, for understanding me and this message and for her commitment to right livelihood and doing the right thing, always.

Allie Rudolph for her vibrancy and commitment to heartfulness and for the inspiration behind the title.

Stephen Levine who first reminded me that the heart can heal our pain.

Kay Mullin who told me food is meant to be chewed and not inhaled.

Foreword for Food Fix

By John Robbins

Author of *Diet For A New America* and *The Food Revolution*, and
Co-Founder of the Food Revolution Network (foodrevolution.org)

Not that long ago, the Beef Council spent more than $50 million on an ad campaign that featured the celebrities James Garner and Cybill Shepherd. The slogan of the campaign—"Real Food For Real People"—was catchy and effective.

The Beef Council was counting on the fact that just about nobody wants to be an unreal person, or wants to eat unreal food.

And yet, if you look at what people are actually eating in this country, you won't see a lot of natural and wholesome food. What you will see is a large amount of food-like substances that pass for food, and that provide instant taste sensations but little true nourishment. And if you look at how people actually spend their time, you won't see a lot of authenticity. You'll see a lot of energy spent imitating and trying to please others. You'll see a lot of people trying diet after diet and still craving low-nutrient foods.

The ad campaign was effective because it keyed into the deep hunger many of us feel to be more real, to feel our real feelings and to be true to ourselves. But there were some rather poignant ironies to the promotional campaign. For one, the path to getting in touch with your real feelings probably doesn't lie in imitating others, even those as famous as James Garner or Cybill Shepherd.

For another, the health of these celebrities was hardly exemplary. Shortly after the ad campaign began, James Garner had quintuple bypass heart surgery.

And Cybill Shepherd later revealed that she suffered from chronic constipation, bloating, and abdominal discomfort during the entire ad campaign and for years thereafter.

The beef council ads were dangerously misleading, but they were on to something profoundly important. There lives in many of us a deep need to become more real to ourselves, to choose real food, to feel real feelings, and to acknowledge and honor the truth of our own lives. And that is where Susan Young comes in, because that is exactly what her marvelous book will help you do.

She shares her own path with naked honesty. She writes transparently about her struggle with food, weight, and body image. She describes in deeply human terms how she has moved toward a genuine relationship with self-nourishment and self-nurturing.

A lot of people realize that our food world is insane, that it's filled with highly processed and artificial "foods" that are toxic to our bodies and our minds. In most cities, it's easier to find a candy bar or a pack of cigarettes than it is to find an organic apple.

In rebellion, in trying to find a healthy diet in the midst of a food world gone mad, you can become rigidly attached to this diet or that one, fervently seeking health with the fastidiousness of a monk. But where does that get you? Do you really need more frenzy and obsession in your life? If your efforts to eat more healthfully are based in fear, your diet may improve temporarily, but will you become the person you are really here to be?

On the other hand, there is the path that lies before you in this heartful offering from Susan Young. It is not a path of more control, but one of more awareness, more consciousness, and more compassion for yourself.

If your steps toward a healthier diet are taken with appreciation for the gifts of your life, if they are taken with true respect for yourself and for others, if they are acts of genuine self-care, where might they lead? Might your life become filled with healthy pleasures? Might your body thank you for the rest of your life?

Foreword

Susan Young is pointing the way, but not to another list of "shoulds." She is pointing the way to a path of awakening and joy. If you listen to your own heart and let her guide you, you may be surprised at what you find.

You may find yourself appreciating your life more than you ever thought possible, thinking real thoughts, enjoying real health, and manifesting real dreams. You may find yourself eating real food, not because you are depriving yourself, and not because you are trying to become a better person, but because through this book you learned how you really, really, really love your life.

John Robbins

Food Fix

Introduction

"What is REAL?" asked the Rabbit.

"Real isn't how you are made," said the Skin Horse,
    "It's a thing that happens to you."

"Does it hurt?" asked the Rabbit.

"Sometimes," said the Skin Horse, for he was always truth-
    ful.

"Does it happen all at once?"

"It doesn't happen all at once," said the Skin Horse.
    "You become. It takes a long time."

— Marjorie Williams, *The Velveteen Rabbit*

My name is Sue. I am a junk food junkie. I can't follow a diet. I have never been able to follow a diet. The good news is that it is not diet alone that will end our struggle with food, body and weight. I needed, we need something bigger than food plans to change our relationship to self-nourishment and self-nurturing—something more whole than counting ounces and grams.

I wrote this book for three reasons:

1. We can recover from needing our food fixes: daily chocolate dose, shots of caffeine, sugar hits, carbohydrate attacks, the munchies.

2. The current obesity epidemic, health crises, and the personal suffering they bring are fixable.

3. Ancient Eastern wisdom teaches us there is nothing wrong with us. From its origins more than 5,000 years ago, one yogic intention is to connect our hearts to something more than just our physical bodies. We will practice this in every chapter of this book, in increments. Simply. You will start to eat the foods that retain their natural

> Although the world is full of suffering, it is also full of the overcoming of it.
> Helen Keller

1

shape and their natural components. The diet that Nature intended our bodies to eat is high in fruits in vegetables and low in animal products and refined carbohydrates. And you will follow Socrates' advice, "know thyself." Through this book, you will come to see that there is nothing in you to fix, because *Food Fix* is more about consciousness than it is about strength of character or commitment to rules. It is more about awareness than it is about being good or getting it right.

We start where we are now, maybe overweight, maybe discouraged, sick of feeling sick, tired of being tired, and then we heal. This book is about the moments in between: the waking up, the ever-present now that connects the past and the future. This passage can feel unreal. Becoming that real person who does not need fixing after all the years is not a quick fix. It can take a long time, a growing up.

As an adult, I became a mental health counselor, teaching master's level counseling students at a local university. I had a private therapy practice for fifteen years. Now, I teach yoga, meditation and mindfulness. Professionally I help people who might be diagnosed with modern eating disorders like compulsive eating, compulsive overeating, binge eating disorder, food addiction, bulimia nervosa or self-starving anorexia.

By 1976, when the song "Junk Food Junkie" became popular, the singer Larry Groce must have understood a not-so-adult non-professional part of me. Like millions of Americans, I had always eaten what normal modern Americans eat: Cheerios and milk, Jif peanut butter on white bread, steaks, M&Ms and ice cream. But normal go-with-the-flow habits of any culture are not necessarily optimal, and by my late twenties I was fifty pounds overweight on a 5-foot 1-inch frame, had hip pain that forced me to quit running, backaches that hooked me on enough aspirin to develop a debilitating lung-congesting allergy to aspirin, headaches that made it impossible to focus, enough indigestion and bloating to pop Tums as snacks and enough self-hatred, paradoxically, to lead me finally to get real with myself. If I used my clinically-trained brain to find myself in any neat diagnostic categories, I didn't fully fit any. But I suffered greatly.

Like the Skin Horse in the *Velveteen Rabbit* whose hair gets loved off and who grows loose in the joints, I grew up eventually. I also had my dark secrets, which I kept especially from people who would not understand. I wished I could have become a real modern girl without being uncomfortable, without changing, without confronting personal and rapid-fire changing cultural patterns.

One secret: I had a long-standing struggle with what, when, how, or even if to eat. For as long as I can remember, I thought I was grotesque when I weighed 175 pounds and I knew I was plump when I weighed 102. I planned clandestine eating love affairs. I chose brownies over salad. I gained fifty pounds. I lost forty. I gained twenty back. I lost twenty-five. When I was twelve, I stole my younger brother's Easter candy. At sixteen, I sneaked out of the swimming pool instead of playing water polo to raid my aunt's cupboard of Little Debbie Snack Cakes. I like, or I used to like, the narcotic-like sugar highs of cheap convenience foods and the coma-like processed-carbohydrate naps. I went through periods of starvation. I went through stages of throwing up what I ate.

Some friends called me a gutter-eater because I took bites from everyone's plate and ate their leftovers, their garbage. "Thou shalt not covet my food," they scolded as they slapped my hand. When Laurie showed me the Vanishing Chocolate Chip Quaker Oatmeal Raisin cookies she had just baked and frozen, I tiptoed to her freezer all day, broke pieces off and ate. They did, indeed, vanish. She noticed: "Susan! You're out of control. Stop."

I couldn't. Another friend called me a designer-addict because for a while I would buy only dark, organic, 80-percent fair trade chocolate at double-the-price health food stores.

> You already have the precious mixture that will make you well. Use it.
> Rumi

I have healed. You can too. I survived and now thrive. You can too.

How? First, we must be clear: this is not a book about helping you fit into a modern-day culturally-approved size four dress by next year's reunion. We need a deeper, more solid intention. We need a broader look. We need to get out of our heads filled with facts of fat grams, ounces of protein and calories. We need to get real, which can seem countercultural. We need what I will call heartfulness, that mature inner place of deep intuition which, when we cultivate its age-old wisdom, knows what is best for us and can lead us to it.

This book will show you:

- There are ancient antidotes to today's screaming food messages. (Remember the potato chip ad, "Bet you can't eat just one?")
- There can be an end to the loud voices in our heads.
- There is an answer to what I'm calling food frenzy, that automatic give-it-to-me-now, I-gotta-have-it craving—that strong desire for the not real foods invented by human beings and made on machines.
- There is a way out. Becoming real and whole happens on many levels. The instructions for healing on all levels are always the same: get real, get simple, turn to the answers that have proven to be healing for centuries.

I'm much older than when I was tormented by food frenzy—when I always lost the fight against the hook to processed, adulterated, bleached, bromated, fractionated foods. I know now that it is possible to overcome food frenzy—those sweet hankerings, those meaty yearnings and unhealthy longings.

Millions of us who do not have a diagnosable eating disorder are haunted by I-need-a-food-fix-and-I-need-it-now; for you, for me, I write this book.

This book is for anyone who:

- even though uncomfortable in our bodies, way too often chows down too fast on too much packaged, processed food.
- loses the focus of our real goal of wanting to be wholly healthy or taking real care of ourselves and has the habit of giving in to "what-the-heck" eating.
- takes a bite, especially if it is soooo fat-sugary-or-salty-tasty, and then wants more.

- pines for "just a little something." We think, "Oh, I've never had this before." Then we want it all. No matter how much we eat, it never seems to be enough.

- feels anxious about food. Do I have the right food plan? Is there a perfect way to eat? What if I never find it?

- can get preoccupied with the minutia of the newest brand of processed foods, the latest promising instant weight loss, the most recent fountain-of-youth supplement, or the method of calculating grams of carbohydrates.

- eats standing up, in closets, in cars, at desks, alone at the television or computer. We gulp, inhale, and don't chew our food. Prone to impulsive recreational eating, with no relationship to physical hunger, we want instant gratification. But we do not want to be seen eating.

- gets started with recreational eating and finds it hard to stop. In the middle of food frenzy, we feel that we have not chosen food—it has chosen us.

> Any intelligent fool can make things bigger, more complex, and more violent. It takes a touch of genius —and a lot of courage — to move in the opposite direction.
>
> Albert Einstein

For those who live with a person caught in the grips of this culture's dysfunctional eating, this book is also for you so you can love the captive in a real way. For those who love those who suffer, this is also for you, so that you can be one who understands. And for those who know they fall somewhere on the continuum between food frenzy and freedom, this book is for you.

This book is not for those who work well with, "I have to be good on my diet today." Healing back into the simplicity of real takes great bravery of stepping into unknown places. Real takes love, to grow, learn and transform away from I gotta-have-it-and-I-gotta-have-it-now. We learn to choose real food, to feel real feelings, and to write, or at least acknowledge and honor, the truth of our own story. This book asks for real work on your part. This book is experiential; it is not for those who want an intellectual formula on how to become. *Food Fix* shows us the path out of food confusion, into a paradigm shift. We learn to ask simple questions: "Is it real? Is it whole?" *Food Fix* offers a change in life

> We don't receive wisdom;
> we must discover it for
> ourselves after a journey
> that no one can take for us
> or spare us.
>
> Marcel Proust

view; it is huge and it is simple and it is what it took for me to change. If I can change, you can, too.

We are a nation in crisis. We spend more dollars on health care than any other nation. We are all prey to the marketing ploys of big agribusiness, which usually seduce us toward one fractionated nutrient supplement (take B vitamins to boost energy) or one part of a food (eliminate fats, or increase fiber, or up the protein). Without the view of wholeness, our overall health declines. Every year obesity strikes more and more adults and younger and younger children. About half of the food we eat is not "real"—quick rice, white pasta, cookies, chips, crackers, soda, cakes, brownies, fast food, junk food—filled with too many calories and not enough nutrition. We are overfed and undernourished. Americans eat only about ten percent of our diet as vegetables and fruits. Half of those vegetables are potatoes, and half of those potatoes are fried. This book is for all of us.

There are (at least) three ways to grow, to transform, to change, or to heal:

1. We can heal or change our feelings from the heart. Much practice is offered in the FIND YOUR HEART antidotes.
2. We can change our understanding, our thoughts and thinking. Opportunities to do this are offered in the KNOW THYSELF antidotes.
3. We can change our behavior or actions. The book offers ideas in the GET REAL WITH FOOD antidotes.

Antidotes to Food Frenzy.

Ancient practices of the heart. You will not heal merely from reading this book. Freedom does not come from intellectual understanding any more than learning to dance comes from sitting in the audience reading a book about the proper rotation of the shoulder in pirouettes. At the end of each chapter there are experiences called Antidotes to Food Frenzy, adapted from five-thousand-year-old meditations from the East. Use as experiments so that you can see what happens to you as you get free from food crazies. It takes lots and lots of practice. Please do the experiments. The first strand invites you to get out of your confused head and drop into your heart where the healing can begin.

1. Find your heart practices begin with approximately one minute in chapter one and build to twenty minutes by the last chapter. Increasing the practice time strengthens impulse control.

2. The ancient art of memoir. The second antidote is my story (and yours in the Antidotes called **Know Thyself)**—memoir pieces that came to me as healing does, not in a straight line, not all at once, but as a becoming. May my story inspire you to get real with your own story. Write it. Speak it. Become.

3. Real, whole foods. So that you can meet the needs of your body, the third Antidote is the actual, physical, concrete choosing of real food, whole food, food like fruit, vegetables, nuts, seeds, whole grains and legumes. Apples rather than apple juice. Brown rice rather than Rice Krispies. Carrots rather than carrot cake. Almonds rather than marzipan. Whole. Real. Simple. These practices are called **Get Real with Food.** Why whole real food? Because if it's not real food, which we need to feed the real cells of our real bodies, we will still require real nutrition, real nourishment designed by nature to nourish our real animal bodies. With fake food, our appetite grows and we keep eating. When we eat real food—plants, Garden of Eden food—we digest it, assimilate it and derive the energy from it that Mother Nature intends. This is the miracle of real. The ancient human body does not know what to do with a list of processed chemical ingredients. *Holos* is the Greek root of the modern English words, health, whole, healing and holy. Choosing wholeness in one area ripples into others.

With all my heart, here is what I know: if you start practicing what is offered in this book, you will eventually create the habit of asking your heart: "What do I really care about?" "What is my real hunger here?" You will get in touch with your deepest intentions for yourself,

Living creatures are nourished by food, and food is nourished by rain.
Bhagavad Gita

7

your health, and maybe even the health of the planet. With practice, wholeheartedness, or heartfulness, becomes who you are. It is a state of being that informs your choices.

> Human beings are set apart from the animals…We may choose order and peace or confusion and chaos.
> Rosa Parks

With our modern, glitzy, newfangled potions, pills, bars and fluorescent packaging, we are eating experimental diets. No one knows if the human race can survive on what we now consume. This book will help you reclaim what you already know because it is wired into your ancient human self: real health, real wholeness.

Begin anywhere. You will get to the heart of your own story. Feed yourself a regular diet of nourishing heart moments and heart-healthy natural foods. You will come to see as I did how these themes of new actions, new thoughts and new feelings are woven together, inter-related and stronger, as in any braid, than when alone. My hope is that you will come to see that the interconnected strands are really no different from each other. To choose one is to begin to choose them all.

The braid of heartfulness awakens us to life. We begin to heal the Whole, the Earth, and our One Body. May you be free of food frenzy.

Part One

Awakening & Getting Real

There is a treasure in your heart.
—Rumi

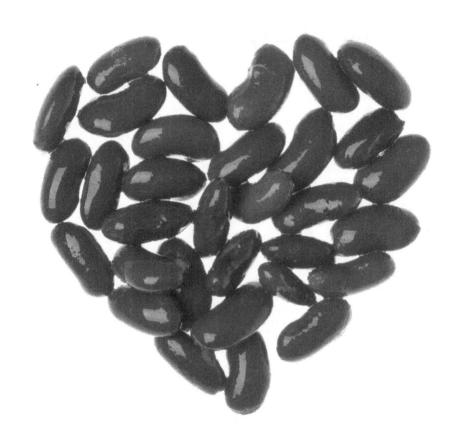

Chapter One

Still Hungry After All These Years

There are many forms of hunger. There is the hunger for food, and there is the hunger for love, for purpose, for truth. There is the hunger for companionship, for inner peace, for the sense that we belong. There is hunger for laughter, and there is the hunger for God.

—John Robbins and Ann Mortifee, *In Search of Balance*

Here's what I have come to know: Feeding our larger human longings invites us into our brilliance and helps us see ourselves in heart-softening ways. Our heart center is enormous. Early and recent mystics tell us that our inner universe is as vast as all the galaxies. Recovery from food hell has to be that big, has to touch our primordial wholeness beyond the knowledge we get from today's books or the newest magazine-cover food plans. It has to be deeper than counting calories, reading labels, weighing proteins or stepping on the scale. Those behaviors can lead to what psychologists call "the paralysis of analysis: analysis paralysis." Reducing ourselves to how many inches our waists measure or how many fat grams we consume each day can keep us "running on empty." Still hungry after all these years. Heartfulness, on the other hand, releases the constriction in the middle of our chests (that feeling of being "up tight"), tames the wildness of the chaotic mind, calms the whirlwind of emotions and puts needed space—heartspace—between a craving, the impulse to fix it and the dive into the food.

For decades I lost myself in Ring Ding cakes and Tootsie Roll candy. Food frenzy, or disordered eating, carries with it anxiety about food. We feel a little crazy. Sizzling barbecued beef, turkey smothered in gravy, juicy chicken with

Bread baked without love is a bitter bread, that feeds but half man's hunger.
Kahlil Gibran

crispy skin, battered fried fish, sugars, processed junk—what dieticians sometimes call "extreme foods" make it difficult to stop popping things into our mouths and to stop obsessing about it. It can be less stimulating, less crazy-making if we remember that we are part of an interrelated ecology, a whole, the planet. Every choice we make either moves toward health for all the systems of our bodies and the world or away from it. In *The China Study*, nutritional scientist T. Colin Campbell, PhD, writes of this integration, "Eating should be an enjoyable and worry-free experience, and shouldn't rely on deprivation. Keeping it simple is essential if we are to enjoy our food. One of the most fortunate findings from the mountain of nutritional research I've encountered is that good food and good health is simple… Eat all you want (while getting lots of variety) of any whole unrefined plant-based food."

Ultimately the antidote to food frenzy is a simple sacred bow to our natural already-given wholeness. If we yield into wholeness, we recover. Because we can't fool Mother Nature, we ignore the natural order of things at our own peril.

I knew this fullness of heart as a child. The primeval ocean taught me. Until I left home as a young twenty-something, I lived on a tree-lined suburban street that wound from my house about a mile to the Atlantic Ocean. Open views of the islands dotting Casco Bay awaited me if I would just visit the end of my road. I could not have put words to my heart's desires then, but I can now, and maybe you can look back at your childhood and begin to put words to your hungers. I know now that I was hungry for how I breathed more deeply at the sea, for the look of the broad horizon, the smell of salty dew, the sound of breath-like in-and-out waves, the feeling under my bare feet as I walked on the steps of the dock, heard the creak of the wooden planks and joined what lie beyond my young world. I craved spaciousness. It was my heart, beating in the center of my chest that led me to the water, and I went often.

I am in high school.

My two-houses-away neighbor Cindy and I concoct special dates to walk to our end-of-the-road pier. We talk about boys and boobs and periods. "Is French kissing really a mortal sin? Will we really skip purgatory and go straight to hell?" As important as getting to the sandbar is, we also feed our hunger for companionship. The weather doesn't matter.

One Christmas morning, after tearing through gifts, I call Cindy, "What did you get?"

She describes a dress—a cream-colored cotton shirt-waist with a rounded Bermuda collar and images of people engaged in various sports in primary colors printed all over. "Me, too," I shriek. "I got the same dress." That Christmas Day at noon, we spiff up in our new twin outfits and trudge through the blizzard to the beach.

In the spring rain, we don our yellow slickers and rubber boots and slosh our way to the end of the road to see the drops hit the waves. On the first warm-enough summer day for shorts, we run up and down the hills of the road, then lie on the old grayish/brown, rickety dock. Feeling the boards sway in rhythm with the tides, we soak up the heat. Our appetites for friendship are filled.

I go alone to the ocean if I feel lonely, which seems strange, being the oldest of seven children. But I can feel alone in the Upper East Side of New York City, and the ocean always welcomes me. I ride my black five-speed English bike to the end of that road during high school, carrying I-will-never-be-loved-again boyfriend conflicts. I entrust this bigness with my first love's announcement, "We should see other people."

Spotting my red eyes and puffy cheeks, Mom comforts, "You're seventeen. Someone will love you again one day."

Dad adds, "And you will love again, too."

But my first love would tickle my chin to induce a smile, had taught me to sail, let me lean against him on the ski rope tow at Hurricane Mountain. Now he would date Kathy. Body sinking, throat closing, belly hollow, heartbroken, I do not reach for Hershey's Milk Chocolate Almond Bars.

> Everyone needs beauty as well as bread, places to play and pray, where nature heals and gives strength to body and soul alike.
> John Muir

The true hunger in me whispers, "Go to where it's big."

I seek Casco Bay's roominess to soften my heart's contracting. No answers come; merely a welcoming presence, holding, cradling, rocking me. I cry. The tides take my tears. I am safe.

I was starved for something I could not name then: a feeling that I did not know until I saw the water, a sense of okayness, knowledge of a mystery larger than me. Sitting, gazing, being still, I loved the assurance of one wave after another lapping the shore. Whether the everyday gentle, almost silent little rippling runners, or the tumultuous pounding remnants of a slapping storm or angry tide, their constancy impressed me. Something always opened up at this outer landscape. I know now that what opened was me, in oceanic movements of the inner landscape. This, if I could only have known, is heartfulness, is home.

> It is not the length of life, but the depth of it.
> R. W. Emerson:

The calm depth of the water spoke to me, no matter what rippled on the surface. The ocean taught me a way to sit in the middle of whatever craziness was in my life, to sit and to wonder, to sit in awe. The ocean taught me the meaning of paradox: feeling whole in the midst of feeling shattered; feeling right in my world when much of it felt wrong. That which is wide, deep and broad can awaken the heart. You might find heartfulness—fullness of the heart—in a green city park, on a hilltop with a broad view, on a walk in the woods. Go there. Feel the expanse, both inner and outer. Notice how, in this real place, troubles can visit and you can be okay.

Rumi, a thirteenth century mystic, wrote:

The Guest House

This being human is a guesthouse,
every morning a new arrival,

a joy, a depression, a meanness,
some momentary awareness comes
as an unexpected visitor.

Welcome and entertain them all!
Even if they're a crowd of sorrows
who violently sweep your house
empty of its furniture.

Still, treat each guest honorably.
He may be clearing you out
For some new delight.

The dark thought, the shame, the malice,
meet them at the door laughing,
and invite them in.

Be grateful for whoever comes,
because each has been sent as a guide from beyond.

I knew as a kid how to welcome sorrows, how to let myself be cleared out, how to trust the guidance of a wide open heart. Then I forgot. As a kid, I ate apples and green beans, raw carrot sticks and celery. I wrote simply in my journal. I played with wide-open heart. With adolescence came TV dinners, packaged pancakes, brownie mixes and the idea that I had to be good, be better, be the best. As the song goes, I looked for love in all the wrong places. I binged. I purged. I fasted. I dieted, followed the popular fads: the protein-only Stillman diet that left me with dank acidic breath; the AYDS candy diet in which I chewed a week's allotted servings of caramels in one sitting (I probably was not sitting); the liquid diet drinks of Metrecal and Slimfast that I stole from my parents' kitchen cupboard; the if-you-eat-only-grapefruit-your-body-will-eat-itself-away diet; Weight Watchers when once-a-week-liver was required and foods were legal or illegal; Diet Workshop, during which I feasted for five days then fasted for two days before the meetings; Take Off Pounds Sensibly (TOPS) where we were forced to wear pink plastic pigs around our necks if we gained weight; Diet

> Beyond a wholesome discipline, be gentle with yourself. You are a child of the universe.
>
> Max Ehrmann

Center with daily weigh-ins and way too much cottage cheese and too many canned peaches.

With both professional and personal experience, I now know that food frenzy is a misguided attempt to fill up on some external give-it-to-me-now. For twenty years my hands grabbed the wrong substances. For decades I wandered along a major detour, labeled myself a glutton, and searched for the road home, which was inside me all the time.

Heartfulness is a homecoming.

Today I live in another house, also near the Atlantic Ocean. Today I take refuge at more power spots by this coast. Now and then I go to one for solitude. Overlooking a busy harbor and bustling marina, one site crowns to a dandelion-spotted bright green hill that slopes down to Casco Bay's panoramic blue. Listening to seagulls caw, smelling clam flats—I inhale salt air—fulfilled rather than feeling full with food. Breathing in, I nourish myself. Breathing out, I feel filled.

Now I go to the water as adult, with all my grown-up hurt that is no less painful than break-ups with high school beaux. The grace of heartfulness, the freely given gift, flowing in every moment, is always available. To benefit from it, I must stop and turn my attention away from the huge forces of food frenzy—the mind screaming how fat and ugly I am (I'm neither), the fear of gaining a hundred pounds, the drive to pop into every corner store. I must claim this inner space.

Heartfulness is both a lifelong journey and the destination, both what we do and what we become. Heartfulness is like walking out into nature. Whereas heartless food frenzy is like hibernating in a claustrophobic closet that chokes us, heartfulness allows us to care for ourselves. The purpose of heartfulness is to show us that we are like the ocean, larger than we know.

The end-of-each-chapter experiments in heartfulness (Antidotes to Food Frenzy) start now and develop for years. They help us break free from our tendency to turn on ourselves, to abandon ourselves. Your engagement in this transformation is what will heal, not the reading, not the theories. At some point, we close the heady books and open the wisdom of the heart. You don't have to do the experiments perfectly: you do have to begin. As in, "you must be present to win," you must participate in an experiential way to change.

Antidotes to Food Frenzy

Find Your Heart (One minute)

After reading this and getting a sense of how to feel into the heart, practice for at least one minute. Turn off outer distractions. Let this be a time of focus for you. Let heartfulness embrace you. Practice after you read this and any time during the day that you can; any time you remember.

Release your weight down as you read this. You may have noticed already that it is easy to get distracted, off track, pulled away from your intention. Our thoughts can get in the way of what we intend ("this will never work"). Emotions arise ("I'm afraid to try"). Physical sensations can sabotage ("I smell the cookies in the kitchen"). Let it all be. Kindly, tenderly, relax your weight down and turn your attention to the heart. With this simple act, you have begun to learn to pause, a needed skill for impulse control.

Heartfulness is traction. The heart can help us get back on track, redirect our thoughts, feelings and actions. Over and over, come home to your center. In the wide sea of heartfulness, let yourself and all your "I-need-it-nows" be embraced, held, supported.

> All things are connected.
> Chief Seattle

Find a comfortable place to sit or lie down. Ideally, choose a place that you can dedicate to these practices as they get longer and longer. Try different areas to see how they feel; a special room, a closet, a corner. Eventually you will have one place that you most prefer.

You can sit in a chair, on a pillow, a bench or cross legged on the floor, or even lie down. Get comfortable. The more comfortable you are, the easier it is to focus awareness rather than fidgeting due to discomfort. Your position is less important than the quality of your attention. The most important instruction is to be able to sit or lie comfortably for a period of time while keeping the spine straight and the chest open. In a somewhat dignified posture, have your spine erect but not stiff, so breath can move freely in and out, which it cannot do if you are slumped and the heart area is caved in. Have your heart unobstructed, sternum slightly lifted as you begin to learn to feel into the body at the heart.

Turn your attention to the tide-like rhythm of your breathing. With belly soft and heart open, see if you can feel into the breath as it comes and goes, allowing it to be as it is without trying to change it. Let it be normal and natural, whatever that is for you, and at the same time noticing what's going on in you as a whole. Stay with what's real, with what is right here in this moment. What can you feel, if anything (e.g., Breathing in, I feel my breath fill my whole body. Breathing out, I relax.)?

Melt into the feel of the breath coming and going to and from your center and allow yourself to feel how you are clearing an oceanic space within. Chest and torso fill like waves coming in, body comes back to center on the exhale. Your thoughts might seduce you away, entice you into planning, or they might judge you. Simply notice your thoughts. They want you to believe they are real; they are only thoughts, and, over time, thoughts change.

Notice, also, how the breath feels. Short? Long? Smooth? Full of static? Feel the inhales and the exhales fully. Even if you feel small and tight, and feel those old feelings of self-disgust or desperation, let it all be exactly as it is. Return to the breath in the center of your chest.

Soon you will practice the above instructions for at least one minute. Stop. Settle. Turn off anything that might distract you during this practice period. Radio. TV. Phone. Close your eyes if that feels comfortable. Stay with your felt sense of the deep heart. When you notice your attention is no longer in your body, simply return again and again, as many times as you need to. Your mind will move away. Each time you notice that you have lost your sense of center, pick up the breath in this moment and anchor again in the deep heart and its wave-like breathing.

At other times during the day: Play with this experiment before you rise in the morning, with eyes open during the day, and again as you fall asleep at night. As cravings arise, notice where your mind and thoughts have taken you, acknowledge where you've gone, and then stop and drop into your center. Any time you think of it, move the energy and attention to your deep heart. Because our old ways of self-hatred, self-judgments and self-destructive patterns are repetitive, we need repeated, daily, committed, disciplines of kindheartedness. Again and again. Over and over.

Continue now for a least one minute on your own.

Know Thyself

Take time to do the reflection now. Put this book down. Your writing is as important, if not more important, than mine.

Write about a time in your life when you knew your own brilliance, your own fullness, your own wholeness. (e.g., the day you learned to ride a two-wheel bike, or when you passed your driver's license test, or cooked your first good meal…whatever). And then write about the possibilities of bringing this wholeness, this aliveness, this being real, into your life now. This work is simple. We already know how to do it.

Is there a way for you to draw an image of how it feels to be caught in the prison of food frenzy? This is not about art. It is about examining the felt sense being trapped in food frenzy. Swirls of color will do. Lines. Squiggles. Use symbols if you want. What comes to you?

Now draw how freedom would look and feel.

The more we feel nourished by whole foods and the whole of our lives, the less we choose physical food to fill non-physical hungers. It is also true that the less we notice the fullness of life, the more we turn to physical food in a misguided attempt to nourish non-physical parts of us.

Explore what has nourished you today. Sights? Sounds? Tastes? Smells?

19

Sensations? Thoughts? Emotions? Conversations? Laughs? A walk in nature?

Start a list in a dedicated journal. (This will develop more and more in each chapter.) This list is to hone your attention, to teach you to see the whole picture and all that is in it, not just that yummy cake in the oven that is calling your name as if it were the only "nourishment" for your soul.

Acknowledge what feeds your non-food hungers. This ongoing, daily practice of "what really nourishes" will help you pay attention. Keep noticing and writing. Some examples follow: Warm water in the shower. The smell of lavender in the soap. A hot cup of tea. The fact that I can sit at my computer because I have electricity. My car runs just fine. Simple. (e.g., Breathing in, I read a loving e-mail from my daughter. Breathing out, I feel nourished.)

> Will you teach your children what we have taught our children? That the earth is our mother?
> Chief Seattle

Get Real with Food

Go to your kitchen and open the cupboards, the refrigerator and check out your countertops. In your journal or on a piece of paper, make two columns. Label one Real Food and the other Not Real Food. Put things like apples, oranges, green beans, walnuts, brown rice, lentils in the Real Food column, put whoopie pies, scotch, French fries, doughnuts, etc., in the Not Real Food list. Without making any of the not-foods wrong, and especially without making yourself wrong for eating them, simply notice the balance of what you have. Heartfulness is not a path of judgment. It is a path of awareness.

Over the next few days, see if you can tip the balance toward more real food and less not real food. Then notice how you feel.

Chapter Two

The Spark Within

Hatred does not cease by hatred, but only by love;
this is the eternal rule.

—Buddha

What does it mean that my big craving took me to the end of my road both figuratively and literally? Just how did heartfulness save my life?

For years my prayer was, "Let me get through this day without snack attacks and food frenzy." Filled with self-hatred, I knew I wanted to lose weight. I knew at least a few danger and trigger foods and, in the moment of choice, I would often feel "what-the-heck" and abandon my best intentions, bingeing on hot fudge sundaes. I threw them up or perhaps merely experienced the automatic sense of self-disgust. "Please, God, if you let me live through this, I vow to be good forever. There will never be a next time. This is it. Honest." I did not know how to practice asking the heart for help and to listen for its sane response.

Not eating never happened. I could never keep my promises because whatever the questions, Baskin-Robbins answered them. And, since "nobody doesn't like Sarah Lee," I depended on her, too. I did not know that I was trying to reduce stress or that I was caught off-balance choosing the Standard American Diet of meats, sugars, flour products and processed foods (interestingly abbreviated SAD). I knew only eating. Boredom led to foraging. Anger relieved by chomping. Sadness; straight to slurping. Discomfort; get the jaw crunching. Heartfulness would eventually teach me to tolerate anxiety, worry, distress and embarrassment without needing a food fix.

I had not yet made the connection that real food comes from real farming. I did not yet know what we now know about nutrition, as outlined by T. Colin Campbell in his manifesto, *The China Study*: "Nutrition is the biologically holistic process by which elements of food and water are brought into the body to optimize health." I did not understand my longings and knew nothing about holistic processes. "What the heck" was familiar, the path of least resistance, an easy quick reaction.

Self-respect buried beneath layered shame, I dared tell no one. What if someone humiliated me? Self-humiliation had already brought me to the ground; I could not survive degradation. Yet, over time, the clandestine grab-the-food/stuff-it-in rituals became scarier and my paranoia escalated. I might somehow be causing throat cancer from toxic foods and a growing habit of trying to throw them up. I convinced myself that I was surely insane. One day, my fear of being found dead on the cold tile bathroom floor surpassed my hot dread of being discovered in the act while alive. I mustered enough courage to call an endocrinologist.

I am in my late twenties.

The lower half of his office walls are covered in rich mahogany, a beveled chair rail marking the paneling's end and pulling my eyes upward toward framed diplomas with shiny gold seals. Undergraduate School. Medical School. Advanced Training. Degrees, certificates of merit, and awards speak of his brilliance. I feel small. The frames all match, thick wood of deep red, meticulously hung in a symmetrical pattern behind his handsome blond head. With a white coat and stethoscope, he sits in a large tufted Chippendale wing chair, the aroma of its soft cordovan leather almost disguising the clinical smell of rubbing alcohol. Distancing him from me is his huge cherry desk, manila charts neatly piled in the corner closest to me. I want to hide.

There are few places where the spiritual, political, personal, and ecological dimensions of our lives meet as fully as they do when we sit down to our breakfasts, lunches and dinners.

John Robbins

Queasiness grips my body. On my first attempt, words catch in my throat. Voice muted somewhat from the lush green carpet, I stumble, "Well... I... er, you see... Um... so, I came because..."

Wholeness includes integrity in our food, which must come from good soil, air and water.

"Mmmmmm?" Drumming his broad, athletic fingers on the shiny desktop, he waits.

All at once, I blurt, "I'm teaching third grade and some days I get so hungry—well, maybe it's not hunger——that I get home from school and, even though I am trying to lose fifty pounds and I know I shouldn't, there is a moment I just give up and say, "what-the-heck." I cave. I eat so much all at once that my heart starts racing and my body gets all revved up. It's so uncomfortable that then I put my finger down my throat and make myself throw up."

Hurried and incomplete; it's the best I can do. I cannot describe the screaming impulses to push anything down, to consume, and to inhale brownies and ice cream sandwiches. I will not tell him about the swirling nausea after devouring, panic that can only be relieved by forced vomiting. In the grips of the perverse binge/purge compulsion, I have been able to explain this to myself. It all seems so logical. Somehow throwing food in and then throwing it up makes exquisite sense in the very moment of despair. No words are available to me.

I can only admit, "I get so hungry... well, I don't have a word for it... There is this moment of going numb, numbing out with food."

He cocks his boyish head and places his bronze cheek on his hand. "Well, what do you eat?"

"Oh, maybe a box of graham crackers with peanut butter and mounds of marshmallow fluff. Or maybe a dozen plain doughnuts, cut in half and toasted with peanut butter and fluff melted on top."

Clearly not the whole truth, even this confession takes guts. I omit the quarts of soft serve vanilla Dairy Queen, used as a dip for a full family-size bag of barbeque potato chips. I don't mention topping it all off with containers of white fluffy Cool Whip. I forget the what-the-heck choice of "Oh-my-God-I-have-to-get-rid-of-this." Simply, some forms of catharsis are easier than others.

First, he strokes his clean-shaven chin, and rubs his tongue along his white teeth. Then he studies a clipboard and I wait for words of wisdom.

His raises his eyebrows. "That's bizarre… good way to give yourself a stroke."

His statement echoes in my head. "That's bizarre? Has he never heard of this before? I really am nuts." Nausea squeezes my gut, the same way it does when I stuff tapioca or Ben and Jerry's that churn inside. I want to throw up his words. I hate myself for revealing to him my deepest secret. Had I been at home now, I would be able to bolt from these squeamish feelings with a trip to the cupboard, then to the toilet. Here in this office, there is no escape.

No diagnosis: he offers a treatment plan. "Well, if you get that hungry, maybe you should have an orange before you leave school."

I told no one. I spent four more years dashing from one store to the next to buy my stash so no one clerk would see all the Hershey bars, kisses and syrups I bought. Four more years of secret terror. Although there were glimmers of awareness of the caving-in moment, of the exact point in time that I abandoned myself, I had no idea about wholeness, about the importance of integrity in our food, which must come from good soil, air and water. I had no idea that I was confusing personal fulfillment with filling up, confusing living with a full heart in the moment for living for the whim of every moment.

I began to devour self-help books, which gave me diagnoses of pathology and prescriptions of what to do. I came to believe I was deficient; many books talked of disease, powerlessness and character defects. At first, the reading helped; I felt less alone. There was a label for what I sometimes did—bulimia. The books reported that the onset of bulimia was often in college; as it was for me. People with bulimia tend to be extroverted, with strong personalities—that's me. Willful vomiting is common in 75-100 percent of people with bulimia. That included me. The books became my friends.

But then there were passages about co-morbidity with depression. That was not me. There were accounts of tooth enamel being destroyed by regurgitated stomach acid; I could not believe this would happen to me. Bingers sometimes committed suicide trying to escape their own frenetic minds; and toilet bowls hosted unintentional suicides. People with bulimia could die of cardiac arrest. Filled with the horror of these possibilities, my mind held a terrible secret. Shame curled my insides into a fetal ball.

> We know so many things, but we don't know ourselves! Go into your own ground and learn to know yourself there.
> Meister Eckhart

When we don't know what to do, we often give up, give in, and revert to old familiar habits. I found a favorite muffin bakery in my neighborhood.

When the mind is clogged with food frenzy thoughts, whether they escalate to bulimia or merely take up residence in our nutritionally-confused heads, the mixed-up thoughts taunt us with, "whatever you eat, it isn't right." Eventually, plant-based eating would teach me that an apple or carrots can never be wrong and that recovery would not be about adopting another diet. Rather I would come to see that, instead of a new food plan, I would need a plan of the heart. I would need, as the '70s saying went, "to give peas a chance." But until I found the plant-based, heart-centered way to settle my inner arguments, I walked alone through food frenzy.

Many of the books offered treatment plans: go to New York for help; gain admission to a three-month addiction rehabilitation program in Florida; get a referral for an eating disorder unit in a Pennsylvania hospital; stop eating sugar and flour; seek out a psychiatrist for medication for anxiety and depression. I was not depressed. I did not want to be on a "unit." Alarm jumped from those pages.

Information alone does not heal, but I did not know that then. Assuming more intellectual understanding would magically cure me, I rooted out more knowledge, grasped outward, and clutched at whatever came along. A little reading from the library had helped a little; a lot from Borders and Barnes & Noble would be better, I reasoned. I kept feeding my head with more books and kept eating what I had been eating. I had no way then to drop into my heart and body for truth.

Happily then, I discovered an easy recipe for no-bake chocolate cookies.

Well-meaning writers, some of whom might have been valuable, only heightened the spiraling inner turmoil. But I kept seeking them, because I thought some authority, someone out there must know better than I did. I wanted to run from these books, but I dared not because some author, often an older male, must have the answers for this young woman. I continued my bulimic relationship with these sources, eating them up, discarding them, grabbing another, throwing it out, and seeking more. I binged with my mind, and then purged the information when it overwhelmed me.

I ate more Fig Newtons.

After the endocrinologist, there were many false starts. I yearned to find someone to trust with my story.

I am in my early thirties.

Shaking, unaware of what I need, I schedule an appointment with a woman, an "expert." As I open the front door, soft pastels—roses and blue paisley on a large upholstered wing chair—an oriental carpet and a vase of yellow and white carnations grace the living room table and greet me. This place looks more like a home than an office; the spaces are light and open. In a casual loosely-fitted dress, a friendly nurse conducts an initial interview at a large, family-size dining room table.

This time I have a name for what I do; bulimia. I feel certain this specialist in this charming environment will relate to voracious appetite, as she has allegedly also experienced not only unnaturally constant hunger but also its harmful compensatory reactions. She would understand these moments of forgetting all we know and choosing brownies instead. I begin to let my bones release down into the soft chair, to feel my muscles let go of their tight holding.

Soon it is my turn to see the professional, my turn to tell my story. Tender sprouts of trust trampled by the return of fright, I, once again, abruptly spew out my words. Bulimic elimination takes many forms; today my speech is staccato, forceful. With the same get-it-over-with quality as a hurried binge, my blurted confession is also the if-I-do-this-quickly-enough-no-one-will-know purge. Fully expecting her to nod her head, "yes," I wait for empathy, for compassion. We are simpatico, I figure, and she is a self-professed healer.

I look at her eyes. I can always see connection in the eyes. She looks at her notes. "Were you sexually abused as a child?"

"No," I answer immediately.

Making "no" with her head, she furrows her brow, and winces her eyes, now staring straight into mine. "Are you sure?"

Annoyed and impatient, I punctuate for her, "Yes." Period. "I'm sure." Period.

I mentally scan my happy childhood. The men in my life loved me. Uncles played cards with me. Two loving grandfathers held my hands as they walked me to the beach and played games with me in the sand. Mostly my four younger brothers ignored me. I felt safe as a kid. I loved my family. As I stood before this inquisitor, flashes of downhill skiing with my dad in the winter and water-skiing behind the boat he drove in the summer flooded my memory. As the oldest of seven children, I was the babysitter. "Yes!" Exclamation point. "I am absolutely sure."

"Well, you may want to look into it. Incest and abuse are very common with bulimics."

Maybe she's talking about herself, I note inwardly, because I do not refer to myself as a bulimic. I think, "I am Sue, mother, wife, teacher, daughter, runner. Sue. In my high school yearbook, next to my senior picture is a quarter-page list of my activities, clubs and honor: President of French Club, Secretary of Student Council, Head Cheerleader, Honor Roll, Softball. Under it all are the words, 'self-confident, proficient, effervescent.' I happen to do this weird, scary thing with cakes, bread sticks and Reese's cups, but it is not who I am. I am Sue."

"If I were you…" she forges ahead although I barely hear her now. I am instead listening to me, the running commentary in my head which is exploring, "Who am I if I not 'a bulimic?'"

"If I were you, I would get clear on my history."

I am clear on my history. I want some relief in my messed-up present. I have come here to ensure my future.

"The best therapist I know for bulimics is in Boston. She is expensive—$150.00 for fifty minutes. Are you willing to drive to Boston once a week?"

"No." Sitting up straight now, I am beginning to feel the first stirrings of a heartbeat in my center. "There was no incest, and I do not want to leave a husband, a one-year-old and a three-year-old. There must be a way to do this work here."

"Well," she sighs, clucking her tongue, "I see you are not ready to help yourself. It's a problem when women don't value themselves. It's also very co-dependent of you not to put yourself first."

No one can make you feel inferior without your consent.
Eleanor Roosevelt

Unwilling to work with me further, not addressing the force of food grabbing and the strong desires that take me over, she is nevertheless more than willing to sell me several bottles of supplements—one to cut cravings for carbohydrates; one to stabilize blood sugar; one to replenish the B-vitamins lost with the stress of the "disease," a special calcium to preserve my teeth, and magnesium for nerves. It does not occur to me that her intervention borders on abuse. But my heart has started to speak and I listen: this doesn't feel right. So I leave.

Today I wonder sometimes, "What is it that kept me going, one rejection after another?" Maybe it's my effervescence. I never stopped questing, seeking to know, to observe myself, to study that precise instant in which I kept handing myself over to the Cookie Monster. I kept moving in closer to this Sue. The heart keeps knocking until we open the door. In yoga classes and on meditation retreats, where lots of fresh salads, vegetable and bean soups are served, teachers point us to our core, that spot around which we can expand into our fullest expression of a posture, of our life. The heart calls us.

Slowly, slowly, slowly I began to pay attention to what I ate and how I felt, to the food I consumed and how my weight was affected, to my nutrition and my lipid profile, to my diet and my moods. Help came, not from books, but from investigating my own experience, as this book asks you to do. When I ate unrefined, unprocessed, plant-based foods, I felt no fear. I felt satisfied, not Thanksgiving Day stuffed. Apples, strawberries, romaine, blueberries, brown rice, lentils landed in me in ways that said, "Yes." My body said, "thank you." The body offers an incredibly wise and intelligent feedback system, which will guide us if we listen; all of me wanted to embrace and not reject whole plant-based foods. When we eat real foods that are in line with our body's natural needs, we also reject ourselves much less. Life's choices are an ecosystem; intertwined.

> The heart wants to be known, to be witnessed, to be embraced... We keep marching toward sympathetic ears.

The heart wants to be known, to be witnessed, to be embraced, and so we keep telling our stories until at least one person hears it… not just listens, but really hears it. We keep marching toward sympathetic ears.

After each wounding it took more energy to reach out again. Several months passed before I picked up the phone, this time to a pastoral counselor. Although counter-productive in many ways, several of the books suggested that the insatiable urge to stuff is a spiritual appetite. A quote by French philosopher Blaise Pascal resonated: "In each of us, there is a God-shaped hole that only God can fill." I called Rabbi Harry. When I married years ago, this rabbi had converted me to Judaism from my native Roman Catholicism. Surely this man would welcome me today as he had when I had studied with him ten years before.

I am in my mid-thirties.

We are to meet in his office. I walk in. He jumps up. Pointing to the door, he announces he has a better idea of where to chat. We walk together into and out of the large, empty sanctuary of the Temple, through a small musty classroom, piled high with dusty books and rickety tables. Finally we sit in a tiny back storage room, the furthest point from any other people in the building. With hardly any space for furniture, we squeeze into the quiet, secluded chamber.

"I think we'll have the most privacy here," he accommodates my wishes without my having spoken them.

As we clunk student-size yellowish wooden chairs across the dusty floor, I do not know how to start, or even why I've come all of a sudden. How can I tell this holy man my profane ritual? Yet I sense we are in some protected inner sanctum in the bowels of this temple. If I bolt from here now, I will only lose my way. And I am lost enough. Somehow the story unfolds. He congratulates me for the courage to tell him.

"That must have been difficult for you."

"Well, yes, of course. It was hard to tell you, of all people. I figured gluttony must be some kind of sin," I confess.

"No, no, that's not what I mean. I mean all those what-the-heck moments of running scared from yourself. That must be very difficult for you."

Blurred together are his words about greater meaning and fulfillment, for they are foreign to me, as is his warmth of heart. I sit here with my first true listener. I lose much of our conversation, but I am able to maintain my posture in the hard, upright, child's school chair with great comfort. I relax. He mentions "seeking behavior." Without a hint of comprehension, I listen as he continues. His gentle acceptance means more to me than his strange talk of inward connectedness and strong currents of desire, none of which I understand. Simply, this feels good. He has my attention now.

He says, "The what-the-heck moments you describe with food are moments of reaching for something. I don't know what you're seeking."

Now I see how I have been expecting these authorities to know. His eyes drift into space, and his focus drops inward. As if having reflected on his own comment, he repeats, "No, I don't know what it is you are seeking, but you do."

I shoot back, "Oh, no I don't. That's why I came to you."

I know nothing but oh-what-the-heck over and over again, and now the rabbi tells me that I know more than I know I know, that I know more than he does. I wrinkle my puzzled brow. "This message is different from all those others," I note inwardly.

"I know there is a Divine Spark in you… in all of us. I think your work is to go inside and get in touch with it. You will not heal by hating yourself. This point of pure truth is untouched by all your suffering."

"Divine Spark? Go inside? What do you mean? How do I do that?"

Opening the top drawer of the old desk, he reaches in with his freckled right hand. When he reveals it again, he has produced a notebook with black and white splotches, a black cloth binding on the left and wide-spaced white paper with blue lines and red margins inside. In high school, we called it a composition book. Sliding it across the weathered wood, he pushes it toward me, "Write."

"Now?"

"Yes. Now."

"Write what?"

"Whatever. It doesn't matter. Write a dream you had last night. Write a sexual fantasy. Write what's on your mind right now. Just write."

Stiffly, tentatively, I write, as if he might take a red pen to it, as if he would care about my sloppy penmanship and careless spelling. He doesn't. He never reads it or questions the content. He wants to know about voice, "what was it like for you to watch your mind like that? How do you feel now that you have written?"

"Watch my mind?"

"Watch your mind. The mind is in every moment and if you get to know it, it will reveal the heart of what is in your habitual, impulsive, maybe even compulsive reach for food. Pay attention."

He assures me that, if I continue to write, I will get to that Spark. Giggling, he discloses that he has filled twelve or thirteen of these books in the past few months. He laughs to think of people reading all his not-holy stuff after he dies. Intuitively I sense he is reaching across our different sufferings to connect. I feel heard.

As if in closing, he adds, "I knew there was something special about you the day I met you. Your spark shone through to me when you were twenty-five, and it shines today. Now you must see it."

I don't believe him. I do believe that he believes himself. His belief in the "center of my being" is enough of a lifeline. I cannot see the heartfulness he sees, but his seeing gives me hope that someday, maybe, I can.

He is not done. "I want you to read something. Go buy a big white book called Healing and the Mind *by Bill Moyers. Read the chapter in which Moyers interviews Jon Kabat-Zinn. That's all. Read that chapter, keep writing. You'll see. You'll be led to greater and greater clarity."*

Antidotes to Food Frenzy

Find Your Heart (Two minutes)

After reading the following instructions and getting a sense of how to feel into the heart in this way, practice for at least two minutes. Turn off outer distractions. Let this be a time of focus for you. Let heartfulness embrace you. Practice after you read this and any time during the day that you can, any time you remember. We increase the length of practice time in heartfulness. As we do, we grow more vitality and vibrancy. Remember to "fill up" even before you get out of bed.

Give sorrow words...
Wm. Shakespeare

Take in these words of Rumi:
Wake up with the morning breeze and ask for a change.
Open and fill yourself with the wine that is your Life.

Repeat this poem. Ask for a change each day on arising and note the changes in you.

Stop.

Breathe.

Feel into the breath.

Feel into the body as the breath raises the chest and lets it fall again. Can you feel the whole body expanding and then returning to center? If so, stay and feel. Soften and explore. If not, get curious, soften and explore. Every time the attention wanders and you bring it back, you strengthen that part of you that can intervene in "what-the-heck." Heartfulness is an inquiry. We have to practice and we have to stop in the middle of those moments of craving so we can choose another action.

Soften the muscles around the breathing apparatus, the chest, the belly, and the shoulders. See if you can let the body be soft. Let the belly be soft and feel the whole body respond to the lungs breathing and the heart pumping. Let the inhales and exhales be comfortable as breath goes in and out.

Let the body fill with air and release it. Soft, easy breaths. Full body breathing. Full body lying or sitting here. Big, like Open Ocean. Heart breaths. Below the turbulence of the waves, beneath the turmoil of thoughts, is depth, is stillness undisturbed by the surface events.

Sit in your deep heart for two minutes.

> Every time the attention wanders and you bring it back, you strengthen that part of you that can intervene in "what-the-heck."

Know Thyself

Now, with this new voice and from your core, imagine telling someone your story. Who would feel safe? Who would both hear you fully and challenge you to grow beyond your suffering? Who will affirm your value, have faith in you, even as you reveal your limitations and obstacles? A doctor? A relative? A support group? A therapist? A yoga teacher? A friend? A clergy member? A dietician? Someone who struggles like you or has struggled in the past? Who? Can you imagine yourself in this conversation? What will you say? How will you ask for help?

If you notice your attention wanders away from the heart as you explore, or if fear overtakes you, simply refocus in your center again and again. This is the repeated practice. Notice what happens. Re-center. Again and again.

Now write this in your journal. Explore the possibility of reaching out for help. You don't have to do it now (many of your old fears may resist this). If you make a routine out of moving into your heart as often as you can, this new habit will prepare you so you can speak from your heart when the time is right.

Get Real with Food

Begin taking action steps now. If you haven't already, start now adding more plants in your diet. Give up on making it hard. Give up on all-or-nothing. You can be imperfect. No matter. Get started now.

Using the image of the heart, one that points you to a whole foods plant-based dietary lifestyle (WFPBD), **make a chart to begin to raise awareness of what you eat.** This chart will also help support you, motivate you and encourage you when peer pressure to eat like others crops up, when you are tempted to say "what-the-heck" or to listen to the voice that wants you to give up on your health. The chart can prepare you for staying in your center when the challenge of being unlike others predictably arises. Draw a heart in the center of the page. Every time you eat a real, whole, unrefined plant-based food, (no added sugar, salt, flour or fat) write or draw it in the center of the heart. Every time you eat a bagel, a cookie, a steak—anything that is not a whole grain, a vegetable, a fruit, legume, a raw nut or seed—write or draw it on the periphery.

At the end of the day, with no judging, only curiosity, note the balance of real food to non-nutritive food. Nutrition for individual and planetary health is a discipline; that is, a training to follow what we know as truth.

Each day, see if you can load up the center more and more with a variety of colorful plant foods. You can use colored pencils as you write in whole, natural foods: purple cabbage, red peppers, green apples, orange squash.

Look at it, study it, get a strong image in your mind's eye so when the urge comes to fuggeddabout whole foods plant-based eating, you can flash on this image, let it pop up and put space between you and your hand-to-mouth habit.

Chapter Three

Beginnings: Fight, Flight or Food

Mental tensions, frustrations, insecurity, aimlessness are among the most damaging stressors and psychosomatic studies have shown how often they cause migraine headache, peptic ulcers, heart attacks, hypertension, mental disease, suicide or just hopeless unhappiness.

—Hans Selye

The word "Meditation" titled the chapter Rabbi Harry assigned to me. My brain skimmed the words of Bill Moyers and Jon Kabat-Zinn about pain and stress-related medical disorders. Yet my heart read the repeatedly stated fact that agitated minds are universal, not problematic in and of themselves. The pages touted the possibility of stillness and peace within difficult situations and emphasized that no matter what, if we are alive, there is always more right than wrong. The words captured me, hit me hard. Stillness. Peace. More right than wrong. What?

Kabat-Zinn wrote:

The mind is chaotic.

I read it again and again.

He did not say, "Susan Young's mind is chaotic."

He did not say, "Your mind is chaotic."

> In the middle of difficulty lies opportunity.
> Albert Einstein

He said, "the mind" is chaotic as if we all share this same mind that loses focus, the same mind that gets off track, fills with unconscious mental activity, and can rant, "What's the matter with me? I did it again. I feel fat because I ate all that granola and I don't want to get dressed because my clothes won't fit and my belly is bloated and I don't want to be seen in public because I weigh more than I did last time I went out and anyway, my midriff bulge will gross out everyone I see and I should know better by now…"

I read that all minds can take off like that. Really? I wanted more.

I felt a connection to all others with this "mind," the familiar jumble in us that can torment us, even if my particular brand of suffering differs. Kabat-Zinn also wrote about our inherent wholeness. He described his work helping people penetrate their pain with awareness, kindness, compassion, empathy, generosity and goodwill. I began to sense the difference between our usual mind-heavy blah-blah-blahs and the lightheartedness that is possible with practice. I could not stop reading.

To not judge what I had called negative and yet move toward more health at the same time provided an answer I had not yet considered. I could put new practices in place when the deep grooves of conditioning wanted to take over. To accept what I hated in myself, to face myself instead of running away, directly opposed what I had known. I knew only what I had heard from a young age from teachers, coaches, relatives, neighbors and friends, which I then installed in my own head:

"Susan, you'll never get a husband at that weight."

"Sue, you have small wrists and they would look pretty if you'd get thin."

> Nothing in life is to be feared. It is only to be understood.
> Marie Curie

"I'll give you $50.00 for a new outfit if you lose fifty pounds."

"You're really smart. Too bad you eat too much."

"Short, fat people like you can only play one position in softball. You'll be the catcher."

I believed them and the voices of the fat-phobic, food-obsessed culture. My mind, an endless screaming cyclone, tore up my inner landscape. Great paradox existed here. I loved my family, felt safe. They loved me. Yet I felt moments of great pain. For all of us, the truth of this complexity pushes and pulls at the heart, that huge place in our core that feels deeply. We must all make sense of the seeming dualities in our lives. We must learn to live out of what we once believed and then live into who we are meant to be.

I turned more pages. Kabat-Zinn spoke of stabilizing the mind and invoking healing energy. Perhaps I could one day learn how to eat and come to terms with what was eating me. This present moment, non-judgmental awareness was called mindfulness. I needed it. New to me yet ancient, these ideas seduced me: we are intrinsically whole; our suffering can be healed (if not cured); we are larger than our pain.

Diets had failed. Restricting calories backfired. Eating whatever I wanted from the candy lanes and the boxed pastry aisle brought a new ten pounds. I had rebelled against external expert advice. Now this chapter promised freedom. The ancient practice of mindfulness could teach us to touch and experience our own essential healthiness, to turn our attention consciously to an open heart and mind, to keep returning to the present moment. I had thought I was crazy. This chapter told me I was human.

I was scared by body hatred, weight obsession, not feeling good enough and never eating right. I read fifty contradictory diet books, adopted conflicting food plans and shared the same misguided misinformation that television feeds all of us. I felt too big, too fat, too short, with hair too straight and too straggly.

Jon Kabat-Zinn wrote that this inner tornado could be seen as a universal tendency of "the mind." I had a brand of what we all have: human suffering. Although this chapter never mentioned food frenzy, the potential of release from its grasp seemed available to me. Mindfulness; that is, paying kind, conscious attention to the present moment, held out a hand to me, a life raft of sanity in a deluge of internal storms.

I do not look sensitive. People see me as "put together." People talk of my high energy and pleasant manner. Effervescent, proficient, self-confident. But I hurt from criticism: criticism from magazines which hinted through their covers and photos that this short, muscular body would find true joy only only if I were stately and blonde as Candace Bergen. Adults repeatedly told me that I'd be happier if I were thin. Boys called me "Tank" or "Fred." Over the years, my favorite way of coping with this inner sensitivity had become a speedy, unconscious connection from the pain and stress of perceived criticism straight to the momentary drug-like pleasure of "treats." As I sat reading the "Meditation" chapter and contemplating whether it was possible for me to change, a flashback erupted:

I am in my thirties.

One Tuesday night, I am presenting the lesson on physiological stress at the Master's level counseling class I co-teach with my friend Reid at a local university. We review the fight/flight/freeze reactions (F/FL/Fr) triggered by the sympathetic nervous system in response to apparent threat. The ancient stress hormones of adrenaline, noradrenalin and cortisol protect our survival by fueling our muscles to punch an alleged enemy, run from peril or halt in place. I talk about how normal F/FL/Fr is, how this hyper-vigilance, with the heart racing, eyes darting, and mind super-attentive developed when our lives depended on escaping from occasional tigers in the jungle. Yet F/Fl/Fr was never designed as a lifestyle, I explain. Since many of us in today's high-speed, high-tech, information-driven, high-pressure, twenty-four-hour-news-cycle world

> A ship in port is safe, but that's not what ships are built for.
> Grace Murray Hopper

live in "sympathetic nervous system overload," we examine in this class how the automatic stress mechanism is over-activated in most of our body-minds. Our stressors might be daily traffic jams, children with prolonged sickness, deadlines. Chronic sympathetic nervous system over-stimulation can keep us stuck in constant, on-going, never-let-up reactions to one twenty-first century blow after another and can lead to anxiety, fatigue, depression, burnout, hormonal imbalances and many illnesses. Fight/flight/freeze. I teach the biology of stress well.

On this particular Tuesday, my usual ebullience cranks up a notch, not seen or felt by me. Body animated, words fly out of my mouth, and I gesticulate with both hands. Bouncing back and forth, I draw such a clever diagram on the board to show how the nervous system interfaces with the endocrine system, how they communicate and affect activities of the whole body. With a big smile, I hand out a piece of paper that has an oh-so-creative cartoon of how the autonomic nervous system has nerves connecting to the organs, the glands and more. "See? The body/mind is integrated. What affects one part affects the whole."

I clearly have passion for this material. After class, Reid whispers, "Sue, you seemed out of your center tonight. I wonder what was going on for you. I wonder if your ego stepped in more than usual."

Reid loves me and trusts me; this I know. Because of our long-term partnership and harmonious relationship, I might safely assume that he wants what is best for the class, and especially what is best for me. Instead I smell danger and my belly clutches in guilt and fear, "ugh, ouch." I am not a fighter, nor do I run. At first, without awareness of my inner stress reaction, I freeze. I cannot take a full breath. Heart racing, tears flood my eyes.

My first automatic thought is, "I gotta have a peanut butter sandwich. Wonder Bread. Jiff. Smucker's."

I am not physically hungry. What I am is invaded by the gotta-have-it grasp of synthesized, processed food, the softer, quicker, and mushier the better. The lightening-bolt connection between discomfort and a sugary-fatty fix happens that fast. For me and for millions of other food-frenzied folks, we need to add another category to the stress reaction pathways. Fight/flight/freeze or food. For many of us, food is our stress management method of choice.

Flashback over, I chuckled to myself that fights, flights or freezes had never interested me. Swift were my food attempts to reduce stress. Rather, I chose M&Ms, Maine-made whoopie pies, Rice Krispie marshmallow bars. I was stuck, entrenched in a mindless habit that cried out for healing.

According to the chapter to which I was now glued, a mindfulness approach to human dilemmas can lower blood pressure, decrease heart rate, bring states of deep relaxation, enhance the immune system and balance the world's over-dependence on progress and technology with inner presence and internal knowing. None of that mattered to me. What I wanted from this fresh approach

Turn toward what
nourishes you.

was far more humble. I wanted my food frenzy to stop.

In food-frenzy mind, the answer to any stressor is food—what to eat or not eat. We seek our fix. Mindfulness offered a rotation in consciousness that would eventually radically shift my relationships: to what I put in my mouth, to how I care for myself and others; and to how I live on this planet. The ground on which I had stood for years began to rumble.

Antidotes to Food Frenzy

Find Your Heart (Three minutes)

After reading the following instructions and getting a sense of how to feel into the heart. Practice for at least three minutes. Turn off outer distractions. Let this be a time of focus for you. Let heartfulness embrace you. In addition, practice any time during the day that you can, any time you remember: Even if it feels uncomfortable, take at least three minutes for practice and skill development today. We need the discipline of strong strategies on which to rely again and again in order to overcome fight/flight/freeze or food.

Right now, stop. Feel into the body. Experience the body. Touch base with the heart.

Attention to breath as filling: Turn your attention to the center of your chest now and any time before you eat anything, even if it's one peanut, or one sip of juice. STOP. Feel the breath. Fill up on the in-breath. Feel its nourishment. Open and fill yourself. If you find it hard to know anything other than physical food as "food," then ask the heart for a change. Go over the "heartful nourishment" list you have been keeping daily and see if you can turn toward what deeply nourishes you. Look at a sunset. Breathe in the smell of cinnamon tea. Listen to Bach or the Bee Gees. Call your best friend. And keep asking your strong heart center to help you open so you can learn to fill yourself with your life.

Ask. Relax and listen into the heart.

This heartwork affects your emotions, which affect your thoughts, which affect your choices of what, how, when and where to eat. Begin anywhere; with thoughts, emotions, body sensations, your own heart. You will heal the whole because all parts are interconnected.

Feel into the breath now for three minutes. Feel into the heart now and whenever you can all day long.

Know Thyself

Pause a moment and ask yourself what you are learning so far. What are you doing to start the change from food frenzy to peace? How is it going? What are you finding most helpful? What still needs work?

Attention to full nourishment: Breathe. Look around you right now and experience what is nourishing. The sun. Summer flowers or new white winter snow. Pictures of your favorite children. The smell of freshly mowed grass or a woody fire. Wind through the evergreens. If it is difficult for you to recognize non-food nourishment, keep practicing. Use your senses. Open your eyes, nose and ears. Breathe.

Find and write at least ten nourishing/nurturing things a day.

This practice stops the food frenzy mind, with all its reaching for what we don't have, plotting to sneak treats when the world is full of them, planning our next binge when we can feast on our senses. Awareness builds over time with repeated and disciplined training. Ten items might take a long time at first, and then you will keep your journal handy as the opportunities to write come to you throughout the day. "My computer works today. I finished the jumble in the paper in record time today. Cherries are in season and delicious. The lilies are blooming and their deep yellow is brilliant. I heard Runaround Sue on the radio today." Like that. It gets easier.

> This practice stops the food frenzy mind...when we can feast on our senses.

Attention to true hunger: In your day-to-day life, begin to pay attention to hunger, physical hunger for food. How do you know when

The student asks: "What is enlightenment?"
The teacher answers: "When hungry, eat. When tired, sleep."

Zen story

you are hungry? What are the signals that you need fuel? How do you respond? What are your patterns? Do you let yourself get hungry? Do you use food like a pill to manage stress? Keeping track of what you eat and how you feel can be helpful.

Whenever you feel "I gotta-have-it," STOP and jot down what "it" is. STOP in the what-the-heck moment and ask yourself if you know what you are doing while you are doing it. Remember awareness and acceptance. What am I craving? Is it food? If I eat what first pops into my mind, will it fill the need I feel? The "I-gotta-have-it" might not be physical hunger or food-related, so we need again and again to let the heart intervene when we hear that voice. We need to pay attention.

Write what you learn about the differences in emotional hunger; impulsiveness and physical hunger.

Instead of fighting the voice and wishing the urges away, running from the body or feeling helpless and freezing, stay with the craving. Breathe. Make space and anchor yourself in your heart. Note your thoughts, body sensations, emotions. See what happens if you write what's happening rather than eat just now. Let yourself investigate. Can you let the craving be there without acting on it just yet? And if you do act on it, how do you feel? It helps to document, as we tend to forget. Be kind to yourself regardless of what happens.

While watching television, list the food commercials you see. Note the words they use. Write them down. Count the ads. Note the bombardment of information from the food and drug industries and big business. Notice if and how commercials impact emotional hunger or impulsivity. How many of these advertisements are for bananas? Romaine? Brown rice? Walnuts? Plant-based dieticians argue that the more dollars spent on marketing, the less nutrition the food likely provides.

Write how you feel after you eat. For example:

"Dark organic 72-percent chocolate bar: jazzed, heartbeat racing, lots of energy for about twenty minutes, then sleepy and a bit jumpy."

"Salad with lots of veggies, corn and black beans, a few sunflower seeds: Feel good, light, not stuffed. Have good energy for a few hours, and then feel real hunger."

Something like that.

We know that stress is the response in our bodies to change. Change can be from the outside (walking into a patisserie and seeing the sweets, feeling the moment of anticipation then some fear). Stressors can be from the inside (the toxic acidic residue left in our digestive tracts after a meat-heavy meal). Since we are an integrated whole and all our choices are interrelated, you will come to see—especially if you document your experiments to help increase awareness—that you feel less stressed overall when you eat whole plant-based foods in their natural state, the way we were designed to eat them. Remember this work is not about "a salad is good." This growth and change are all about awareness.

Get Real with Food

Imagine, or have before you, a peanut butter sandwich. White bread, with any creamy, sweet, commercial brand of peanut butter, and jelly (or, if you'd rather, any processed food will do).

Also imagine, or place before you, the whole plant foods from which this processed food originated many steps ago. Peanuts, grapes, apples, strawberries or raspberries. Imagine or see them on a plate.

Attention to reactions: Staying aware of your heart center, look at the sandwich (or the artificial food) and notice what happens inside you. Do you want to scream and devour? Are you drawn to it? Repulsed by it? Do you want to dive into it or pull away? What do you feel inside? Simply notice. Does the heartbeat quicken? Do you feel any fight/flight/freeze stress reaction? You may feel nothing. Whatever you feel is what you feel. Note it. Are you still sitting in your heart? If not, can you return? If we wake up to how we feel and look deeply into our foods, our choices change over time. Be gentle.

Then imagine or turn to the whole plant-based foods, the ones you have put in front of you exactly as nature provided. Do the same practice. Stay. See the food and feel into the body to see what happens. Do you want to move toward it or away from it? Do you get a "yes" in your core or a big "yuck?" At first, plant-based whole foods do not offer us the same kick, the same jolt or jazzed energy of sugar-laden, caffeine-enhanced, salty, fatty addicting stimulating processed foods. Simply notice how you feel inside as you look at the plate.

Attention to Cravings: The first step in healing or in change is always awareness. The next is acceptance. First feel into the heart area. Breathe. Settle your attention in the middle of your chest. Feel into the body. If you are hungry and you want to, eat what you have chosen and then notice how you feel. Notice your thoughts about yourself. Notice how you feel and notice how the body reacts. Sit. Breathe. Notice. Get inside these pushes and pulls that can ruin your day if you fight, freeze, flee. Stay in close to what happens in your center (find it again, return to it again and again) after you eat. Practice moving closer to the heart, staying close to the heart, feeling into the heart of a craving.

Get to know the nature of the cravings that claw at you. They arise and pass, if you let them, without grabbing for food so quickly. The irony is that when we eat real nourishment that sustains life, cravings diminish. Try it. Eat an apple and see how you feel over the next few hours. Then, at another time, drink apple juice and wait a few hours to see how you feel. We can learn to pause when we feel cravings, feel them, let them be and consciously choose how to respond rather than react with numbed-out food frenzy. Over time, this new habit intercepts and derails the automatic fight/flight/freeze/ food reaction.

Attention to positive stress hormones: We know now that "tending and befriending" is a beneficial stress response, especially for women whose hormones naturally bring us into relationship. Women release oxytocin, sometimes called the hormone of love and bonding, under stress. One of its many functions is to stimulate uterine contractions for labor, bringing a mother into relationship with her child. If we are under stress, the release of oxytocin makes it more likely we will pick up the phone, call a friend for tea or a walk. Let this naturally-occurring "befriending" response be an option when you fall into the old habit of thinking junk food is your friend.

> Befriending ourselves is the start of this process.

Prolactin is another stress hormone that is released and stimulates milk production when a mother hears her baby cry (a stressor). This causes the mother to feed her baby. When prolactin is released due to tension or fear, we move toward others. We are wired for connection and, under stress, if we seek these bonds, if we "reach for our mate (or any other "befriending") instead of our plate," we can heal the myth that food fixes anything. Befriending ourselves is the start of this process. Breathing in, we smile. Breathing out, we smile. We soften our hearts toward ourselves as a stress reliever. We can write a note to ourselves or to another. We can gather, talk or laugh.

Keep plenty of fruits and veggies ready, cut-up and easy to grab. Try adding a salad a day and see how you feel. Next time you are hungry, stop and see if it is physical hunger. If it is, can you eat a plant? Real physical hunger will lead you to real physical food. If you do not seem to want real plant food, then ask again if you are truly physically hungry. It might be a different hunger. Begin anywhere, but begin. Try a salad. Choose an apple. Dip carrots in hummus. Since your behavior affects your thoughts and your emotions, you can start with choosing food to nourish the brain that runs your life. It's all connected.

Trace and then write the steps in the development of the processed food you put before you. Is it factory-made? Where do the chemicals come from? For example: Smucker's Sweet Orange Marmalade's ingredients are high fructose corn syrup, corn syrup, orange peel, orange juice, fruit pectin, citric acid,

> Our food choices have an incredible impact on the initiation, promotion, and reversal of disease, on our energy, on our physical activity, on our emotional and mental well-being, and on our world environment.
>
> T. Colin Campbell

natural orange flavor. What are they? What do they do in the body? How are they made? Where do they come from? Can you go to the source? How are they, or are they not, a match for human nutritional needs?

Trace and write the source of the real food, the peanuts or strawberries. Where do they come from? Can you see the workers, the growers, the pickers, and the people who had a hand in this plant food? Can you feel its connection to the earth, to the elements of air, sun, water, soil? Write your awareness. How was the food grown? What does this whole plant food do in the body? Can you begin to see what real foods do for us? Let what you discover help you choose more real food each day. How can you deepen and broaden your perspective on the value of having a body? Work to understand the importance of taking care of your body and nourishing it in a certain way.

Chapter Four

Eating Heartfully:
We Are How We Eat

The control of the palate is a valuable aid to the control of the mind.
—Mahatma Gandhi

I was ready.

Having read one short chapter, I now knew a few things about mindfulness. Newly popular in the West, mindfulness calls us to an old perspective: the mind and body are not separate, a concept that dates back 5,000 years. I had learned in thirty pages that mindfulness has to do with being fully human. It seems Eastern—i.e., less about scientific or industrial progress and more about learning how to live in harmony with oneself and one's world.

With my interest piqued, I wondered if these ancient technologies could strengthen that Spark. Would mindful living and eating stop the dieting, breaking diets, restricting fats or carbs or sweets, bingeing, rebelling, making up rules, breaking them, all to sabotage my own health, which I so wanted to improve? Committed to learn the answers and to cultivate inner calmness, stability and insight, I decided to try an exercise offered by Jon Kabat-Zinn. He suggested the simple act of eating one raisin. "No problem," I thought.

I am in my late thirties.

I close the book and immediately face my first encounter with a mind clogged with doubt and confusion, a restless tsunami. Do I take an organic jumbo raisin, which means I'll get more substance? That also means more calories. Or do I take an organic golden raisin, which the book has not directed me to do? My turmoil could really mess up this experiment. Generic non-organic, basic SunMaid raisins sit on the top shelf of one of my kitchen cupboards. On the cover of the bright red box, a smiling maiden holds a bounty of grapes and raisins surrounded by a lovely yellow orb. The happy primary colors on the outside seduce me, but I worry that the chemicals and pesticides on the dried fruit inside the package might kill me. I don't know how to continue.

My mind wonders, what should I be doing? Oh, yes, paying attention to the present moment. I'm supposed to open to the experience of eating. But I can't make this first simple choice. My gaze scans the shelves for other options, then darts around the room desperate for something else to do, anything else, maybe alphabetize the spices. I remind myself to chew, to taste, to feel the movements of my tongue, and to feel the texture of the raisin.

Before I even begin, I'll-never-get-this-right and I-will-fail-again fill my head. I choose the jumbo. I like volume.

"The point is to become aware of the moment-to-moment direct experience of eating," I remind myself. I continue, needing to tell myself again and again to stay present in the present and to the present without judgment. Right here. Right now. No right. No wrong. Simply feeling into the body. Mind spinning, I know at least that raisins constitute real food, plants meant for human consumption in the natural order of things, unlike the 12-ounce bag of milk chocolate-covered malt balls I used to choose. I go on. I remember all the raisins shoveled in over the years, all the handfuls eaten robotically in the past. What's more, old food rules in my head project "This won't work" into the future. After all, I am about to eat between meals. I'm not hungry. I'll get fat.

One learns by doing a thing; for though you think you know it, you have no certainty until you try.
Sophocles

With past fiascos and future fears colliding, my scattershot thinking keeps me from staying present.

Back to the book.

Eating Heartfully: We Are How We Eat

Sitting to eat, everything in me speeds up. I cannot let my weight down fully in the chair. I can't sit still. I get up. I read the book. I jump up to get water. I bolt away from the table. I open and close the cupboard. I don't know why I can't settle, and none of this hopping around makes sense. An engine revs in my gut, my mind whirs, and I feel a press to go fast and finish this excruciating raisin-eating exercise.

Then my attention ricochets back to the chapter.

The idea is to chew, and to notice. Finally I sit and pick up one raisin. Pea-size, it falls soundless into my hand, dances around in my palm, opaque, shiny reddish-purplish-brown jagged rows and ridges, the valleys more darkened, the peaks reflecting the light. The raisin has a tiny little stem on one end of its oval shape, evidence, perhaps, of once being connected to something larger. I roll it between my thumb and forefinger. Plump, puffy and squishy, it yields to the soft touch. I can nevertheless feel the bumps, the indentations, and the rough, shriveled texture. The dry sweet smell of the raisin tickles my nostrils as my arm, knowing exactly where to place it, lifts it to my nose to smell. I write in my journal:

Salivating begins.

Craving arises.

I want some.

Now.

I put the raisin to my ear,

hear Rice-Krispie crackling.

Anticipation builds

as my arm places the raisin precisely

in the mouth,

on the tongue.

Dry and cold on the outside,

it smooshes.

My teeth silently crack it open

with the knife-like ridges on my incisors.

> It is not because things are difficult that we do not dare; it is because we do not dare that they are difficult.
>
> Seneca

> Let food be thy medicine
> and medicine be thy food.
> Hippocrates

Sweet, juicy on the inside,
a taste explosion,
a burst of sweetness.
I chew.
One big jumbo raisin.
Taste buds want more time with this delicacy
but the tongue,
like a tiny broom sweeping,
shoves it to the back of my mouth,
as if to hurry the gulping along.

A nurturing miracle exists in this little sun-kissed natural morsel. I acknowledge the sun, rain, soil, earth and wind, all part of this plant food. The growers, the harvesters, the farmers all contributed. This food can sustain life because it comes from life, not from a factory or a chemistry formula like my M&Ms. This is real.

This one raisin contains the whole universe: seeds, grapes, the elements. Body and mind relax somewhat with this real-food, real-life, real-plant realization. Nevertheless, I notice I want to swallow way too soon—even before I stop chewing. Turning this raisin over in my mouth, the muscles of my tongue push it back toward my throat for final consumption. Without warning or explanation, I freeze. Everything stops. My throat grips and clenches shut.

The chapter doesn't say what to do with body tense and jaw tight. This is clear: I do not have my own permission to nourish myself. I want to flee. Armpits sweaty, heart pounding, all muscles contract. I do not understand this inability to nurture myself. I am afraid to eat. I never knew that. Tears trickle down my cheeks as I sit with the impossibility of allowing, of receiving, of nourishing. Never before have I eaten consciously, slowly like this because this act of sitting at the table denotes that I deserve to be fed. And I don't.

The motor inside me kicks in now and I choose the fight mode of the stress reaction, madly throwing down raisins by the fistfuls, as if the tossing will blast through my blocked esophagus, handful after handful, as if the unconsciousness will unfurl my tightened gut. The old voices move in, sneakily at first, then with more might. How do I resist that familiar cry, screaming in my head, "Come on, eat. Susan, don't be ridiculous. Get a grip. It's just one damned raisin."

This place in the eating scene is where I usually give up, "I will never do this again." But this time, another deeper voice speaks, too, one that is even older than the voice of shame. It has been here all along, since before I could talk, no doubt. I had not been able to hear it. In the far reaches of my mind, I sense very faint words, which I am just beginning to know as those of the heart. "Stay present; do not abandon yourself to that old habit." That refreshing whisper fans the Spark, strengthening it in the midst of what Zorba the Greek called the full catastrophe of living.

If I can pay attention now, when I least want to, if I can open to this pain, and breathe some space around the tears, if I can practice with real, plant foods, which feel safe and a match for the human animal rather than eating the extra fudgy brownie mix from the box, I will learn something. A lifetime of mindless consumption shows itself in this one raisin. I see my rejection of the raisin and my rejection of myself through years of autopilot eating. "Healing will come," the heart voice beckons. "Stay here with yourself. I will teach you how to say 'yes' to what really nourishes. I will teach you how to say 'no' to the blaring ads for junk food that would derail you, and I will help you learn to let go of the fear of devouring everything."

I had fallen upon heartfulness of eating—the bringing together of mind, body, feelings and real, whole plant foods at the place of the vulnerable heart. I knew I must now learn to live with courage (as in *coeur*, the French word for heart). It would take a constant re-tuning, returning to the sustaining, nourishing words of the heart and nourishing foods offered by nature. But I had begun.

Antidotes to Food Frenzy

Find Your Heart (Four minutes)

After reading the following instructions, and getting a sense of how to feel into the heart, practice for at least four minutes. Turn off outer distractions. Let this be a time of focus for you. Let heartfulness embrace you. Practice any time during the day that you can, any time you remember.

> The uplift of a fearless heart will help us over barriers. No one ever overcomes difficulties by going at them in a hesitant, doubtful way.
> Laura Ingalls Wilder

Awareness of how it feels to sit with food: This time, get a whole plant-based food, as it grows in nature: an apple, a carrot, a banana, squash, spinach, a tomato. Repeat what we have been practicing. Sit with it. Breathe. Breathe into the heart.

Feel your center. Focused awareness can inhibit automatic thoughts and habits and reduce impulsivity. Practice anchoring your attention in the heart again and again. Look at this real food you have chosen. See if you can both notice this food and feel into your body at the same time. At first, when we turn to real sustenance, we might miss the buzz from sugar or the coma that follows chips, burgers and fries. Sitting with food might feel new if you tend to "eat on the run" or "grab a quick bite," or stuff your face at the fridge. Choosing to eat well leads to more choosing to eat well and the process unfolds over a lifetime as it uncovers and releases old habits. The foods we take into our bodies become our bodies, so awakening the body to how we feel pays great dividends. When you sit with food, notice how you feel about receiving it, letting it in, allowing yourself to be nourished by it. Can you sit with food and also receive the breath? Can you feel receptive to what the heart will teach you? Can you open? Get curious.

Awareness of what's going on before you eat: Stop before you eat this whole, real food, if you do decide to eat. Are you hungry? First practice taming the need for instant gratification. Pause. Breathe. Notice. Feel.

Before you take a bite, stop, center and feel into any emotions: mad, sad, scared, glad, bored, embarrassed, ashamed, disgusted, loving… whatever, open to it. Feeling any signs of fight/flight/freeze or stress? Breathe. Come back to sitting in your heart again and again and bring the open, kind qualities of the heart-mind to this inquiry. Heartfulness reduces stress and reducing stress reduces gotta-have-it impulsivity and makes what-the-heck moments easier to navigate. All of this happens only in the now, in this moment, not next Monday, not New Year's Day. Practice being free of food frenzy right here, right now. It will strengthen you for the moments to come.

Awareness of what's going on as you eat: If you are hungry and want to eat, then do. Notice what happens. Do you savor? Devour? Enjoy? Taste? Smell? See the color and texture? Do you clutch at food and eat faster and faster? Do you let yourself feed yourself without shame, guilt or fear? Can you bring joy to the act of nourishing yourself? Feeling bad about eating can lead to more eating. Simply notice. Keep moving into your heart and keep paying attention.

Know Thyself

If it helps you, keep writing what you eat and how you feel. Write what goes through your mind. Write about your emotions. Write how your body feels. The heart can accommodate all feelings, so if you feel scared, stay with fear. If you feel happy, embrace happiness.

> [We] go abroad to wonder at the height of mountains, at the huge waves of the sea, at the long courses of the rivers, at the vast compass of the ocean, at the circular motion of the stars, and [we] pass by [ourselves] without wondering.
>
> St. Augustine

Keep up your list of ten healthy pleasures every day. What nourishes your soul and spirit? This practice will help you come to value that which fills you. Identifying what you do right nourishes, too, so write your own strengths. Like this: "Today I took a strong walk for an hour." "Today I sat in silence at the bedside of my sick mother." "I managed to clean all the kitchen cupboards today." Give yourself credit.

Acknowledging our assets empowers us to make good choices. Writing them down helps us remember them later when we might otherwise fall back into old mind patterns.

Make a list of changes. If you do not now eat in a way that you would like to eat, write how would like to eat. What would/could you change about how you eat that would support your overall wellness? If you have goals, write them. See them. Breathe them in.

Keep noticing and keeping track of how you respond or react to hunger and cravings. Do you experience how hunger and cravings differ? Pay attention to the subtleties. Note, too, as you eat more and more plants that these nutrient-dense foods feed you so well and fully that you crave junk food less: when the body is nourished with the elements, minerals and nutrients it needs, you will make wiser decisions. When we give the body what it loves, the body-mind loves us back. Can you let food be one of many options of how you receive nourishment? Do you eat to fuel your body or do you eat recreationally? Notice. No judging. Simply stay aware as much as you can. Documenting it can help.

Get Real with Food

Awareness of the whole: Real food, Nature's bounty, cannot be outdone by synthetic chemicals, supplements or processed foods. Heartfulness touches our whole being. Whole plant foods transform how we look and feel, as these foods address whole nutrition needs.

Sit and feel the whole of you. Breathe and feel your whole body. For four minutes, simply notice what's nourishing and nurturing around you. (Later, note any ripple effect during the day.) See if your exploration of heartfulness grows in you, gets easier, and notice if you can trust your inner wisdom more and more. Does more compassion flow from you, to you and toward more compassionate food choices? Heartfulness, when practiced regularly, changes your relationship to food, your body, your life and the world.

Chapter Five

Leaving Home to Find Home

You can never cross the ocean unless you have
the courage to lose sight of the shore.

—Christopher Columbus

Clutched by the failure of the raisin experiment, I sat at my homey kitchen table, alone. What, in this experience with simple fruit, had derailed me? I set the intention to investigate this agitation and to wind my way back to my heart's innate goodness. Awakening the heart, having the mind be one with this larger awareness, could hold powerful healing, learning and answers. The process was dark and excruciating.

My mind began to wander, to wonder, and to play with this idea of the inner heart spark. What I came to call heartfulness challenged a core belief that had bossed me around for years: "There is something wrong with me." Coach Smith told me I was too uncoordinated to play basketball. Dad told Professor Hearle I ate too much.

The messages from my new teachers offered antidotes. As I sat contemplating the words of the chapter—they bore their way in, like a long swirling line curling, curling, curling toward my heart. In the midst of this reflection, a flashback of my childhood family dinners popped onto the screen of my mind.

I am eighteen.

I am not sitting. Rather, I jump; the charge of mealtimes bolts through me like a battery, compelling me to be in motion. I am the oldest, Mom's loyal, capable, and willing assistant. I am blonde-haired, freckled-faced, the slightly chubby tomboy who wins neighborhood hula-hoop contests, plays kick-the-can after dinner, draws hopscotch on the beach, and gathers Gretchen, Mary and Janet for gymnastics shows on the jungle gym.

There are nine of us, unless Dad has had a hospital staff meeting and will eat later. Seven children. I have arranged the chairs on the green and yellow plaid carpet, set the table, folded pastel paper napkins into a pocket to hold the stainless forks. My four brothers laugh, make faces, fight over placemats which encroach on each other's territories, and grab one more onion-covered browned pork chop from the serving platter. One of them screams at Mom, "I do not want applesauce touching my mashed potatoes."

Every night another brother spills something, usually knocks his milk over, and with scrunched shoulders pouts as he pounds the table, "I do not like this recipe for banana bread."

A third brother protests, "I hate peas. I have always hated peas. I do not eat peas."

A fourth brother jokes, diverting attention. One of my sisters is quiet. The other rushes to finish in order to make a dash back to the barn and her Appaloosa. Before sitting down, Mom portions out plates for the entire family, demanding every bite be eaten or no dessert—a packaged angel food cake, a Betty Crocker brownie with harlequin ice cream, red Jell-O with gobs of Cool Whip or sometimes, in the summer, watermelon slices. Handsome Dad sits with us, often humming Louis Armstrong tunes and strumming his fingers. Mom serves. Each night she mumbles under her breath, yet audibly, "everyone else is done before I even get to the table."

Only her after-meal cigarette, held delicately in her fine long fingers with manicured nails, and black coffee with exactly two drops of skim milk, calm her agitation. I smell the smoke. I bounce up to get more juice from the refrigerator, wipe up Paul's spills, swipe Mike's peas from his plate, chuck them, answer the phone, and clear the dishes. My place is at one end; if there can be an end to an oblong table. Short and round myself, I belong at the rounded corner nearest the counter and the kitchen work space so I can maneuver, leap up to get a clean fork, and replenish the family-style plate of raw carrot sticks and cucumber rounds. I am the closest to the sink, so I can put the pots and pans in the warm sudsy water.

I eat. I even get seconds but I don't land. It is as if the chair has an electric jolt and, as my butt meets it, my whole body catapults back up. If I can just be good enough, maybe suppers could be more peaceful. If I can be the best helper, there might be more family harmony. Whatever it is that keeps me afraid to sit, the rush that takes over my body barks orders: "Run. Jump. Move. Get busy. Stay busy. Do not sit still." I obey. Mind shuts down; feelings unavailable to me, I am driven by this wired chaotic energy. It feels normal.

I do not ever—even as a kid—feel at home at the dinner table. Too much to do; too much "Poor Sue, too bad she's so chunky. Too bad she can't eat these DQ Dilly Bars like the rest of us." Because I therefore cannot give myself permission to receive, as a teenager I steal the chocolate and vanilla ice cream sandwiches from the refrigerator, sneak into the upstairs bathroom, as far away from the kitchen as possible. I never tell anyone where I am going, where this sweet cold creamy stuff will keep me company. I close the door behind me, lock it, sit in the tight corner on the closed plastic cover of the toilet, smelling the minty Crest drips on the Formica counter, and furtively and repetitively shove the contraband into my mouth. I squish the wrapper inside the discarded toilet paper cardboard, throw it in the wastebasket and cover the flattened tube with the still-fragrant empty Dial Soap box. Although I'm on the second floor, I guard the view from the window to make sure no one can see me. I don't remember if anyone ever did, but I'm sure my secret vices were no secret.

Back to the book chapter and the raisin, a lifetime of suppers appeared. I chastised myself as plump all over again. I did not allow myself to eat, even after all these years as an adult, even after losing fifty pounds. Terrified to swallow, as if not ingesting could keep the memories from cascading, I saw that, as food enters the mouth, it drags along its "feeling" baggage, attached to every emotionally-laden bite. When we most need our own hearts, we are often sitting in our heads in judgment, digesting old material. Like most of us pulled into food frenzy, I was unhappy, self-loathing, ashamed, and trying to keep it all secret, bingeing in private.

I sit again with the one raisin. "Where is this calmness and stability of mind, this human instinct toward healing, that Jon Kabat-Zinn offers as a possibility?" I ask myself. My arm trembles. The intention in this exercise is to savor one raisin mindfully, but, after the frenzy of stuffing myself with half the box and after reliving family dinners, when I start again, I can not raise my arm to my mouth.

Before me in the present moment is the adversity of the past, which can pull mightily on the now. Mindfulness teaches, "The past can invade the present. Pay attention." Native Americans have a proverb, "Don't let yesterday use up too much of today." I breathe and decide to try again.

Can I muster the courage (coeur-age) to stay this time, not run to my bathroom? The mind settles a bit. I start to pay attention to the heart Spark. Can I stay present with this one exercise? I want to stop the inner war, but my very being is the battlefield.

The chaos in my head and the outrageously severe battle of two voices continue:

"Susan, there is so much to do. Hurry and get this stupid raisin-eating thing over, so you can check it off your 'to do' list."

"No, wait. There is nothing to do right now. No place to get to."

"Oh, come on. What's the matter with you? You can be using this time much more productively. Don't you have to call Dr. Savage to make your next appointment?"

"Oh no, there is no place to go right now, nowhere to fly off to. This is very important work. I am starting to sense the value in facing this onslaught, and

the energy it takes to stay with it. Stop. Breathe."

"What do you mean? No radio? No paper? No TV? No magazines? No phone? No conversations? What are you, crazy?"

"That's right. Just eating."

"How selfish of you. Look how much time it takes you to do this, when you could be folding laundry, ironing, or maybe clipping coupons. Shame on you."

"It's okay just to eat. Nothing else. This food is simple, real, and delicious, and I don't want to miss it."

"Just think of how much time you would lose if you ate like this all the time."

"I want to sit and feel what it's like to be in my own body experiencing nutritious plant food without jumping up or out of my own skin as I have my whole life."

"Susan, this is ridiculous."

"I am now relaxing and enjoying my raisin. It is okay to nourish myself."

I chew the raisin and find me. Eating real plant food in peace, I begin to end the war or at least leave the battlefield. I sense that I will be okay, even when feeling afraid. Sitting, breathing, chewing, feeling the sun, rain, wind and soil in this natural food, the Spark's ember becomes a flame. The flame opens up more internal space. I bring the agitated mind to the heart. The raisin eating exercise ends.

This awakening of the heart, this invitation to perceive ourselves more kindly, creates breathing room, a space of possibility and imagination. We begin to see ourselves with what I now call Big Heart. We experience hunger in new ways. We know more about what is real, in whole plant food nutrition, in real foods and in the compassionate heart where the flame resides. This is heartfulness. Ultimately, the healing of food frenzy requires us to let go of any obsessive daily commitment to finding the perfect supplement, to eating the perfect protein bar, to being thinner, to how we look. Healing is much bigger than any of that.

Over time, I came to see that being healthy and whole had nothing to do with dieting, wanting to look young forever or vanity. Health had everything to do with a commitment to the heart's divine spark.

Antidotes to Food Frenzy

Find Your Heart (Five minutes)

Turn off outer distractions. Let this be a time of focus for you. Let heartfulness embrace you. In addition, practice any time during the day that you can, any time you remember.

Stop.

Sit.

Breathe with your whole body, especially around your big, wide, spacious heart.

Move your attention to what is happening here and now in your heart area.

Breathe into the center of your chest and let all the muscles around your breathing relax so the belly rises and falls with the chest as you breathe in, and falls as you breathe out. Can you feel the whole body breathing out from that deep center?

Breathe into your center.

Feel the heart at your core. Anchor yourself here.

After getting a sense of how to feel into the heart, practice for at least five minutes.

Ask this deep heart what kinds of food would deeply nourish you. What foods have enough life force in them to bring you alive? You do not need a book for this. Your body-mind knows. Go to your heart, the place in you that enlivens and enhances us.

Ask.

Listen.

Stay for five minutes. You might think you are done before that. Stay. Even

> Peace comes from within. Do not seek it without.
> Buddha

if you feel restless, expand your capacity to grow. Listen into the heart a little longer. Soften as you enter the heart. Explore what's here again and again.

See if you can find a picture of your early family at a meal or eating. If you can't find a picture, imagine it in your mind. Notice feelings that arise in you. Does the picture trigger fight/flight/freeze or wanting more food? How do you work with this stress? Are you using the practices of dropping into the breath, feeling into the heart, dwelling in the present moment, staying here for a bit more time each day?

Know Thyself

Try an experiment. Write your name. See how it feels. Notice ease, comfort or tension, whatever. After you are done, write your name again with your non-dominant hand. At the same time, note how it feels. Most people report words such as "awkward, messy, feels like I am in first grade."

> Never interrupt someone doing what you said couldn't be done.
> Amelia Earhart

Yes, of course.

When we do what we do automatically it feels familiar. When we try a new idea, it can feel like a problem. We can feel like a failure. But if you kept writing with your non-dominant hand, over time, it would feel more and more comfortable. That is how leaving your childhood home to find your own home can feel. Stay with these practices until they become more and more the habit you choose.

Write or draw what your dinners looked like as a kid. Meat and potatoes? Creamed corn? Macaroni and cheese? Know that if you ate this way for twenty or more years, then there is likely a blueprint in you, a visceral patterned template of beliefs, emotions and habits that might feel as if it is dictating to you today what constitutes a meal. Your early childhood imprints and your ability or lack of ability to eat the way you want today are not separate. Even with your best intentions to eat vegetables, fruits, whole grains and legumes, even with the latest science on plant-based nutrition, even as you think maybe today you'll try almond butter and raisins on hearty spouted bread, your mind will take you back to your emotional bond to the buttery grilled Velveeta cheese on Wonder Bread you had when you were ten.

> Traditions that have lost their meaning are the hardest of all to destroy.
> Edith Wharton

What was home? What is home now? To become fully who you are, you need to be aware of when and where to leave the values of your childhood home—maybe changing favorite recipes, maybe altering certain customs, maybe rethinking inter-generational patterns. You must become your own authority.

Be gentle with yourself as you try a few meals of all plants and then see how you feel. Write it so you can go back to it and recall any differences from when you ate a meal of steak and fries (after which I fall asleep), or a huge salad with lots of colorful veggies and a few beans sprinkled on top (then I feel light and energetic). See what happens when you rethink what nourishment is.

Load up your plate with as many colors as you can.

Go back to what you learned at family suppers. Because of old "What's-the-matter-with-you, what-are-you-crazy" messages, and because of the way the human mind works to try to protect us, you might believe you are messed up. You aren't. You are confronting old patterns and habits. What we used to think can gnaw at us (pun intended). This happens to all of us as we grow up and out of our old homes to find our true home. Do you have a belief that you have to do all the cooking? Do you have a belief that it's your job? Do you believe you can change this? These old voices may never go away, but with practice, we see them more and more for what they are and we don't let them boss us around so much, nor do we believe them quite so naively.

> Rather than what you think you should want, discover what you really want.

Rather than what you think you should want, discover what you really want. Rather than what you learned you should feel, what do you really feel? Can you do this without guilt? If you write in your journal now, you can look back later to see how you're changing.

The full nourishment list: Can you list twenty things right now that nourish you? Pause and do it now. When you see the yellows and golds in an amazing sunset, savor them, appreciate them, let yourself experience these moments of your life instead of rushing by them. Let them fill you.

> In everything give thanks.
> 1 Thessalonians 5:18

Try speaking your list or one or two things on it with one or more people today. See what happens when you say your gratitudes out loud. Often when we acknowledge how full we are with life's abundance, our hearts warm toward ourselves and others. Try it and see.

Get Real with Food

Try this practice with mealtimes. See about serving family style from a buffet or an island or even on the table. Prepare really colorful food, lay it out and let people decide what to serve themselves. If

> Gratitude is not only the greatest of virtues, but the parent of all the others.
> Marcus Tullius Cicero

someone wants something you did not prepare, let that person prepare it. If you want to have black beans and brown rice but others want meat, see about starting a new practice of letting them buy what they want and let them also cook it. This way you do not have to be a "good wife" or a "good girlfriend" or a "good husband." You choose from the same basic ingredients and each person gets what he or she wants.

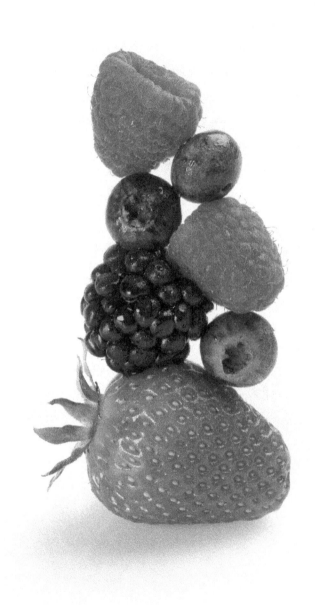

Chapter Six

Self-Compassion

You can search throughout the entire universe for someone who is more deserving of your love and affection than you are yourself, and that person is not to be found anywhere. You, yourself, as much as anybody in the entire universe, deserve your love and affection.

—Buddha

At the beginning stages, my first mindfulness teacher was this one chapter in Bill Moyer's *Healing and the Mind*. Jon Kabat-Zinn wrote that breath is nourishing, in and of itself. It provides life force energy and oxygen to the cells. Without full vibrant breathing, and without self-compassion I would now argue, we cannot live well. I had tried to have a flat board for a body. I had sucked my stomach in for more than twenty years. I wanted no curves, no belly. Breathing freely would push those abs out. Not acceptable. No breath. No self-compassion.

According to the meditative traditions, breathing nourishes deeply, and provides a place of focus in order to train the mind to be calm, a place where we can let go of judging ourselves. Running from corner store to corner store to stock up on penny candy and then driving from pharmacy to pharmacy to buy laxatives are the exact opposite of calm and self-compassion. I hungered for new ways to nurture myself, so I stayed at my kitchen table after the raisin-eating exercise to see if I might deepen my experience of mindfulness, self-acceptance and the flow of breath. Breathing in, I felt cool air in my nostrils. Breathing out, the air was warmer. Trying to allow space for this kind, nurturing breath, I

65

puffed out my belly and chest with one big inhale. Again, memories I had been avoiding for decades flooded in with the in-breath. After chugging a glass of water, I let out an anxious gasp, and was thrown back to my first college dorm.

I am eighteen

It starts innocently enough. We are first year college girls—called "freshmen"—accepted into a prestigious school. Bright. Going places. I attend both high school and college in the 1960s, a time for women to feel big, a time for expanding our horizons and our view of ourselves. Our mentors and role models teach that we are not going to be "just housewives." The world is ours.

These are the days before co-ed dorms. We are eighteen- and nineteen-year-old girls, away from home for the first time, hanging out in the hallway in our plaid flannel pajamas, giving each other haircuts, giggling and gaggling the way girls gaggle and giggle when boys aren't around.

"Did you hear about this awful disease Bobbi has?" someone asks one night. We live in the south dorm, Bobbi lives in the north. None of us know her, but the word has spread.

"Her father is a famous internist, and even he can't figure it out. She has to eat four or five platefuls of food every night because something happens to her after meals. Almost immediately, her food throws itself up. She can't keep anything down. She has to get back to the dorm really fast after dinner in order to get to the bathroom before vomiting starts."

When I hear this, I think there must be something terribly wrong with Bobbi's esophagus, or that maybe she has bad reflux, or excess stomach acid. None of us has ever heard of such a disease before, so I stare at Bobbi the first time I meet her and later when we pass on campus. I expect her to be wasting away. She isn't. Her weight seems normal in the face of what I assume must be devastating malnutrition. But she never looks happy, and I simply assume it's because she has some pathology no one can name and that she is probably dying.

I don't have a faulty esophagus or a malfunctioning stomach, but the idea of being able to throw up food that feels uncomfortable sounds like an incredibly creative idea. In the '60s, young women have been made big promises, encouraged to lap up life, drink in all the possibilities, to chew up and spit out the patriarchy. The energy being fed us is enormous, and we are having our consciousness raised so that we can devour it all.

We are still digesting the messages from the women who raised us; women who watched their dads weather the Great Depression and stood by their men through World War II. Our mothers are women who started families when the veterans returned. They are women who themselves had been trained to be homemakers. Our childhood homes showed us how to serve men dinner. Before we escaped to this dorm, we watched our mothers sit down last. They taught us to clean house and to iron. We went to church, no questions asked. But our 1960s culture worships at the altar of idealized thinness and the perfect body, whatever that is. Despite the protests of the new feminists, "Stay home and care for others" is what we learned at home.

I did not notice, in 1967, the tension that these opposites set up in my cells, but now I am aware that, for at least a decade, I never took a deep breath. Deep breathing might have helped my angst, but when anxiety squeezes like a vice grip around the heart, self compassion gets squeezed out and panic sets in. I had been trying to fix fear with food. Breath went into my brain, I suppose, which was working hard to compete at this school. Unconscious to the dilemma which bound me, I had no conscious way of nurturing myself through it. Unknowingly, I was caught between two generations, between two worlds. But my body knew the pull of these polarities, and not breathing long breaths became the automatic physical stance which held me in whatever tenuous balance I could manage.

We sit in the long corridor of first floor South night after night. Mary says, "Thank God we're not sick like Bobbi, but did you know, I heard once that if you swallow a teaspoon of yellow mustard with a gallon of water, then stand on your head, hold your breath, have someone hit your stomach, and then jiggle around, you can make yourself throw up after a big meal?"

Mary is from California. That's how I figure she knows these things.

Some of my friends quit at this point. But four of us think this technique of dealing with discomfort is brilliant. I, for one, see this as the perfect answer to my constant quest, "How can I do it all?"

Of course, there was more to food frenzy than I knew—perhaps more than I will ever know. Analyzing reasons only in the head can be misleading and not always helpful. But somehow it makes sense to me now, when I ask the heart, that bingeing and purging were my best answers to that part of me that was wondering, "How can I simultaneously be a perfect take-it-all-in woman of the '60s and a perfect daughter from the '50s?" Perhaps food frenzy, and by extension bulimia, are inspired adaptations to a confused society. From the heart's point of view, I was doing the best I could, given what I knew at the time.

Anna, Mary, Karen and I gather all the glasses we can find, fill them with warm water—it had to be tepid water—steal a commercial-size yellow plastic jar of French's plain mustard from the senior dining hall, and hunt down a teaspoon. Here we are, past lights out, assisting one person—who has to be holding her breath—to do a headstand. The helper's job is to hike the feet in the air, while one other person rubs or punches the stomach of the upside-down girl, and everyone works at jiggling her all at the same time. Next is a race to the bathroom, where the idea is to push an exhale. Then we wait for the vomiting.

Nothing happens for me when I am upside down, except for dropping some loose change. I hate mustard. Its pungent smell tightens my nose and squints my eyes. After these ordeals in the hallway, now I loathe mustard, and, even with my protruding stuffed belly, I never throw up. Even with no hope, still, I pile my plates higher and higher at dinner to prepare for this ritual, but I have no luck. I cannot get the trick to work.

Over time, my fellow experimenters lose interest, and fewer girls show up in the hallway. But something intrigues me about the possibility of over-filling my-self with whatever processed food I want and then being able to get rid of it, as if the body had never received it. As if there would be no consequences.

In my field of mental health counseling, this extreme rationalization might be labeled a cognitive distortion, or perhaps irrational thinking. But it didn't feel wrong at the time. Body image was at stake. Success in higher education was crucial. I can't explain exactly how I made it OK to continue as if bingeing and purging were perfectly normal, but I did.

Awareness deadens during a binge. I numbed a body that was judged by society as too fat, too hungry, too short, with too many desires. With total lack of self-compassion I had taken those beliefs as my own. I made Dean's List every semester and graduated with high honors yet had no body intelligence. I had no idea when I was physically hungry and no signal to stop once I started eating, especially if it was cheeseburgers with fries, milk shakes and maple-walnut ice cream. Junk food might satisfy a sweet tooth or a craving, but it cannot lead to accurate body signals.

No, yellow mustard and four quarts of water never works for me. But then Sam from Boston tells us about using a spoon to tickle the back of the throat to induce vomiting. No one mentions another word after that, and I don't know who keeps trying and who gives up. The lure of getting all that I want of goodies, treats, sweets and Wonder Bread concoctions—and not gaining weight—propels me. Now it is my secret; not even my eating buddies will continue. It is getting too weird, they say. I keep going. I am driven.

The spoon begins to feel like a skeleton in my closet. I hide it. It haunts me. I hide myself and go to the bathroom alone now. I drink the gallon of water—belly wash, someone calls it—but I never get it right. The spoon only scratches my throat and I throw up nothing but blood.

As in school, choosing a major that excites me, dating a smart boyfriend, and feeling happy with my friends and skiing. If anyone asks me, I say I love my family. I love my life. It is true.

There is also a desperate me. How can I be part of this expansive liberal arts environment? How can I take advantage of all it promises? How can I think big, and stay wide-eyed? How can I go home fifty pounds heavier to four fit brothers, two skinny sisters, and parents who criticized me for being too fat before I left? I am afraid of my old neighborhood, where people had clucked their tongues my whole life, "It's amazing that you look just like your father. Too bad, you're even built like him. Solid. Football player type. What a shame you're not more like your mother. She is so thin and beautiful."

Now I weigh what my father weighs.

I am trying to make sense of being eighteen, smart and female. I am trying to be obedient to everyone, no matter how inconsistent. I am trying to comply with every cultural norm in the late 1960s, no matter how confusing. Into the culture come Rice-A-Roni, Fiddle Faddle, Pop-Tarts, Fritos, Tang and Hi-C. Processed foods proliferate. Without the awareness and self-love to see things clearly, I eat them all.

Not only are the reasons for what I am doing unknown to me; food frenzy itself has an unconscious quality to it. Shovel fast. Don't feel.

I ache from hurting myself with dangerous non-nutritive substances and treacherous behaviors. Performed with reckless abandon, these actions close the heart in on itself. We shut down in shame carrying tremendous guilt and fear.

In college, nightly, before the Student Union closes, I make a nine o'clock run for Vermont homemade chocolate chip ice cream, French fries, chocolate chip cookies and coffee with half and half. Slurping it until way past stuffed, each night I then decide that chocolate chip ice cream is not quite the right flavor. I need the chocolate for sure, but something seems missing so I order a large bowl of Cherry Chocolate Chunk. After I devour it, I take a jumbo dish of Strawberry Berry Delight to go—just in case. In case of what, I never ask. Wanting to die of embarrassment if caught, I buy Borden's cherry pies from the filthy vending machines in the basement of the dorm and Toblerone bars, swished down with Pepsi, from the campus bookstore. Every time my friends and I walk into town to do laundry, I eat a giant loaded pizza from the deli next door to the laundromat. We drink Boone's Farm apple wine. Many suppers consist of three puffy white dinner rolls stuffed until they ooze with creamy peanut butter and purplish raspberry jelly. On the days I ski, lunch is a large hot chocolate with melted marshmallow and a thick, chocolate-chip-filled brownie.

And now I sat, all these years later, trying to breathe, trying to overcome the shame of the paunchy belly that muffin-topped over my belt when I took a deep breath, trying to sip water for nourishment. I couldn't forget how I used both breath and water for a college weight loss trick. When I finally found self-compassion at the table that day reading Bill Moyer's book, simple breathing seemed all I could ask of myself. I closed the chapter and sat for six minutes.

Antidotes to Food Frenzy

Find Your Heart (Six minutes)

How long can a human being go without food? Weeks? A month?

How long can we go without water? Days?

How long can we go without breath? Minutes at the most. When we are out of touch with the truth of the heart and our real human needs, we can fool ourselves into believing the pushes and pulls of appetite. We can forget to drink water and we rarely appreciate our breath.

For now, sit for six minutes. Sit. It will help with impulse control.

Breathe. Feel into the breath in your center. Come home to the heart. Anchor in your core.

Notice how the breath is nourishing, how it is nutrition for the cells.

Feel the pleasure of oxygen fill you.

Slow down the breath. Deepen the exhale. Exhale from your deep heart.

Sit as if your life depended on it. It might.

Feel the pleasure of relaxation on the out breath. Let the inhale fill the heart. Fill up on life-giving air. Notice when you bring attention to the heart, it seems to rise in the chest, makes more room.

Sit for six minutes whether you want to or not. Sit with as much self-compassion as you can. Sit for practice. Sit for training. Sit as if your life depended on it. It might.

Know Thyself

Write about how your eating has changed over the last two decades.

Update your Self-compassion list: List all the things you are doing with whole plant-based foods that are right. A salad a day? Two fruits for breakfast? A baked apple before bed? Two servings of veggies at dinner? Trying new types of fresh produce for the first time? Trusting yourself more? Whatever it is, list it, so you can see your progress and practice being kind to yourself.

Write what is working, what you feel good about and any specifics about how you feel a bit more freedom from food frenzy.

List one pattern that you would like to release. Can you write from your heart, with great compassion for where you are right now? Write what you think would happen if you let go of this one habit.

A grateful heart sits at a continual feast.
Proverbs 15:15

Keep your list of what's nourishing every day. Today, try pausing every time before you eat and write or note ten to twenty things other than food that nourish you. See what it feels like to say a few of them to someone else today. A grateful, full heart does not reach for junk food. According to Proverbs 15:15 "A grateful heart sits at a continual feast."

Look over your food charts, if you have kept them, to see how you are changing. Are more and more real plant foods being added to the center of the drawing? Can you start over again each time you eat in a way that takes you off center? Can you start again without beating yourself up, or better yet, with great self-compassion?

Get Real with Food

Now get a big glass of water.

Sit here with it.

Breathe first.

Take a sip.

> I've learned from experience that the greater part of our happiness or misery depends on or dispositions and not on our circumstances.
>
> Martha Washington

If you pay attention, can you feel the nourishment from this life-giving source? Can you take a few deep breaths and a long drink? When we appreciate alternative forms of true nourishment, our cravings for junk subside.

Beginning when you awaken and before 6 pm, every hour on the hour, sit, take a long drink and feel it nourish you. Feel into the body. Breathe and drink. Feel the nourishment from the elements of air and water.

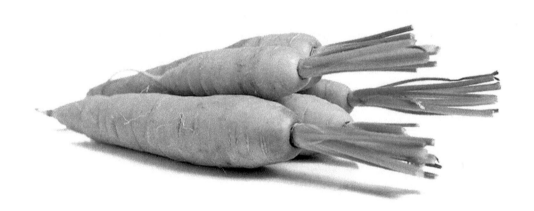

Chapter Seven

Don't Go Back to Sleep

The breeze at dawn has secrets to tell you.
Don't go back to sleep.
You must ask for what you really want.
Don't go back to sleep.
People are going back and forth across the doorsill
where the two worlds touch.
The door is round and open.
Don't go back to sleep.

—Rumi

I read Jon Kabat-Zinn's words again and again that first morning. Eager to learn, I re-read that chapter, "Meditation," many times. It was sweltering outside; ninety degrees and humid. Even as I read and studied, a sweet-tooth craving for Ben & Jerry's Chocolate Chip Cookie Dough gripped me. My new heart-opening skills and heart-friendly foods, which would one day envelop me, were no match for this insistence. I was not, by reading alone, awake or creative enough to transform the craving, or non-violent enough to take good care of my nutritional needs. I had to have ice cream.

At the doorsill where the old and new worlds meet, I had been lingering that morning. I would go back and forth for a long time.

The corner store was only five houses away, but I was in a big rush to get the object of my desire. I jumped into the Grand Cherokee, mouth salivating as I anticipated the moment, in the not too far future, when I would have my fill.

Cool, creamy relief only seconds away, I bombed down the hill, the store in sight now. Ice cream would provide the perfect nutritional snack: protein from the milk, fat from the cream, carbohydrate from the sugar.

DAMN! No parking spot. Food frenzy escalated, my senses in a state of heightened arousal. "I gotta have this ice cream fast." I parked the Jeep, blocking the fire hydrant next to the gas station directly across the street. I ran into the store, formulating my strategy. "Go straight to the cooler, find the flavor, don't look around to be distracted by anything else, pay, jet back to the Jeep. Eat."

What's this?

No!

No Chocolate Chip Cookie Dough? I saw an array of colorful Skittles, Milk Duds and Junior Mints. I wanted something else. The scent of pepperoni pizza slices wafted through the shelves and counters. Like an addict whose supply had been cut off, I felt the impulse to grab as much as I could. I started to sweat, my heart raced. My mind whirled. "I need. I want." If I went next door to the next store, gratification would be delayed too long. So I hunted for another flavor, chocolate the only real requirement.

Peanut butter cup ice cream. I snatched the pint and paid—exact change. Quicker that way. I hopped into the car and slammed open the glove compartment door to find the plastic tableware hidden for just such emergencies.

The black leather interior sizzled in the sun. I turned the key to start the air conditioning, and I began to coax the embedded peanut butter cups from the solid vanilla base. I noticed that the needle for the gas tank had fallen to the left, reading "E"—a good thing, I reasoned. I could sit and eat this treat right now, right here at the gas station pump next door, while Sean filled the tank.

"Fill it up, please."

Imprisoned by unconscious numbed-out actions, I continued to gouge the ice cream. Tough work. In the frozen creamy hardness, those little bits were bricks, stuck as in mortar. It became a battle of wills: I was determined to scarf this down; the ice cream did not melt. Occasionally one rock-hard Reese's chunk jumped out of the pint onto my tan shorts or onto the gray wool runner at my feet, on the floor of the Jeep. No time to clean it up; I was on a mission. Crazed, my jaw tightened, my fist hacked away, and the mining for peanut butter cups accelerated through the hard unyielding white mass.

Now my khaki shorts sported sticky stains all over, beige cotton T-shirt splotched with drips. The perfectly-fitted removable floor mat held puddles of melting white blobs. The steering wheel felt tacky all around. I chipped away. I needed my fix.

"Ahem… Mrs. Young. Er, uh… that'll be $20.45."

Lifting my eyelids from my digging, I saw Sean standing outside the driver's side window with the little black plastic credit card holder, offering me his greasy skinny black ballpoint, waiting patiently for me to sign the receipt. Unaware of my speed until this very second, I cringed at being caught. How long had Sean been there? How much of my shoveling into the pint and slurping had he witnessed?

With "hand in the cookie jar" guilt and shame, I shrugged my shoulders, squiggled up my face, and without making eye contact, offered, "I was hot."

Raising his eyebrows, Sean uttered, "Mrs. Young, can I ask you something?"

In an attempt at nonchalance, I answered, "Sure."

"Are you eating that ice cream with a knife?"

My eyes darted opened. My chest pounded. I wanted to hide. Instead I froze. Until this instant I had not noticed that I had been stabbing this unmoving concoction using a small white plastic knife with serrated edges. Even if I invented a story, the uniformly spaced rake-like grooves in what remained in the colorful cardboard container would have given me away.

I *was* sawing away at a pint of ice cream.

I stopped this time because Sean stared at me through the window, his face inches from mine.

"This is it," I vowed. "Enough. I am done with this pattern."

It might seem trivial compared to other binges. Just one pint of Ben and Jerry's paled against my intake yesterday:

7:00 AM: one chunk of 100% baking chocolate, a small box of dry Raisin Bran, one two-quart bag of popcorn, one peanut butter-flavored THINK RIGHT protein bar, one box of wheat-free, fruit-juice sweetened oatmeal chocolate chip cookies.

10:30 AM: one pint of Soy Essence frozen dessert, another protein bar.

Noon: A one-quart size bag of rice crackers, dipped in and finishing off a pint of tofu/blueberry pudding, one piece of organic dark chocolate.

4:00 PM: Two cups of chocolate soy milk, one bar of halvah, one slice millet toast, one small bag of Veggie Booty Rice and Corn Crackers.

7:00 PM: Large Bag of corn chips, handful of Wheat Thins dipped in Starbuck's Coffee ice cream.

Not one vegetable, not one fruit, no whole grains, not one real meal, not one bite eaten at a table. I did not at the time see this as abuse. I saw it as choosing fats, proteins and carbs. It was only the next morning when my body offered nausea, bags under the my eyes and exhaustion, before I got out of bed, that I could see this as food-hangover.

In the middle of food frenzy, we are not awake to the truth: we can't tell craving from hunger; we don't know filling up from feeling fulfilled; we can't differentiate between a need for mental stimulation and a cup of coffee; we don't know whether to take in a deep cleansing breath or to inhale a brownie.

It did not matter that yesterday was textbook pigging out, this one small pint of Peanut Butter Cup Ben & Jerry's served as a moment of awakening for me, a strange epiphany. I came to want something greater, something more creative, and something less violent to my system, than this habitual behavior. In this embarrassing moment I resolved, right there on my sticky car seat, to follow a path that would open and expand my heart. I committed to learning how.

So it went in those early days of opening my heart. There were moments of great awareness, of commitment-making, then a major falling off the path. Eventually I would recognize the "heartlessness," acknowledge the digression, and start over.

Now, many years later, so it goes. There are moments of feeling awake, aware, connected to the heart, and alive. Days of eating raspberries and walnuts for breakfast, vegetable soup for lunch, brown rice and lentils on a huge colorful salad for dinner. There are still moments of forgetting. Today, the difference is a growing awareness and then the ability to return to the resolution to awaken to something more nourishing, more filling—again and again and again, moment to moment to moment.

When my physical body is hungry, I am awake to its need for food. When the energy in my body needs attention, I can take a few breaths, or a quick walk. When my brain needs "food," I can choose a good book or an inspiring conversation.

When we focus on wholeness, we can awaken to the truth.

> The breeze at dawn has secrets to tell you.
> Don't go back to sleep.
> You must ask for what you really want.
> Don't go back to sleep.
> People are going back and forth across the doorsill
> where the two worlds touch.
> The door is round and open.
> Don't go back to sleep.
>
> —Rumi

> ...this is the noble truth of the end of suffering: it is the complete stopping of craving...being emancipated from it.
>
> *The Pali Canon*

> This seems to be the law of progress in everything we do; it moves along a spiral rather than a perpendicular; we seem to be actually going out of the way and yet it turns out that we were really moving upward all the time.
>
> Frances E. Willard

Antidotes to Food Frenzy

Find Your Heart (Seven minutes)
Stop. Breathe into the deep heart.

See if you can read and receive these words and the words of the poem above from your heart, not your head. Part of the work of heartfulness is to learn to drop our energy and attention into the heart so we can make decisions from our center. First we learn to breathe into our core. Then we learn to spend more time there.

What we practice expands, so cultivate deepening your awareness, nurturing greater balance and ease.

With your feet firmly on the ground, notice the heartbeat, if you can.
Feel the breath.
Feel that you are a whole human being.
For seven minutes right now, feel and breathe into the body.

Know Thyself

The Full Nourishment List: To add to this practice, if somebody irritates you, or things don't go your way, stop and say or write ten things that are nourishing in this interaction. If you fill up with life, you will navigate your cravings with the heart of self-compassion rather than your stubborn old habits. Your expanded full nourishment list might look like this:

First we learn to breathe into our core. Then we learn to spend more time there.

My friend doesn't call when she says she will: I get to practice patience. I get to sit still and breathe. I get to get up and get a big glass of water. I have time to write in my journal.

My vegetable stew burns on the stove; I get to practice how I handle not getting what I want and how to deal with getting what I don't want. The sun is setting…

Begin to think in categories of real foods. Have I had fruit? Have I had whole grains? Have I had legumes and beans? Nuts and Seeds? Have I had root vegetables? Leafy green vegetables? Flowery ones like cabbage and broccoli? Have I had an array of color? Purples? Blue? Oranges? Reds? Each of these "food groups" gives us a variety of phytonutrients, fiber, antioxidants, minerals and the micronutrients we need to thrive. (See bibliography for many books which offer the science of whole foods plant-based nutrition; see also the section for low fat, whole foods, plant-based recipes.) The heart is aligned with nature. Real food is aligned with nature. When we eat a variety of whole plant-based foods, we get all the macronutrients we need. It takes reminding ourselves again and again. A re-minding.

Start today to write your food in color. When you eat blueberries, mark them in blue. When you eat purple cabbage, color it in purple. By the end of the day you will see how varied and nutritious your food is. If all the colors are white: ice cream, white bread, salty chips, items made with Crisco, not only will they all be outside the center of the food circle, your body will be craving real food. Track a few days and you will see. Remember, this is not about good or bad, right or wrong. We are learning to strengthen the attentional "muscles" to keep us on track with plant-strong choices, even when old habits try to pull us away.

> The right way is not always the popular and easy way. Standing for right when it is unpopular is a true test of moral character.
> Margaret Chase Smith

List 10 reasons that it is important for you to choose plant-based living. What are the advantages for you as you wake up to a plant-based whole foods diet? Don't go back to sleep!

> Lunch kills half of Paris, supper the other half.
> Montesquieu

Get Real with Food

Load up a plate of colorful plant food and then sense it, smell it, see the colors and textures, feel how it feels in your mouth. Know that this wholeness includes the metaphoric and physical heart-healing qualities of whole plant-based foods. This awakening to heartfulness means letting go of food groups like fats, protein and carbohydrates. When we think in those categories, we can fool ourselves into believing that ice cream is good for us. After all, ice cream has all of these macronutrients.

Observe your nourishment and your response. Breathe with what you discover. Savor. Enjoy.

Part Two

Returning Home Again and Again:

REAWAKENING

Come
Come, whoever you are! Wanderer,
worshipper, lover of leaving

Come.

This is not a caravan of despair.
It doesn't
matter if you've broken
your vow a thousand times, still

Come,

And yet again, Come.

—Rumi

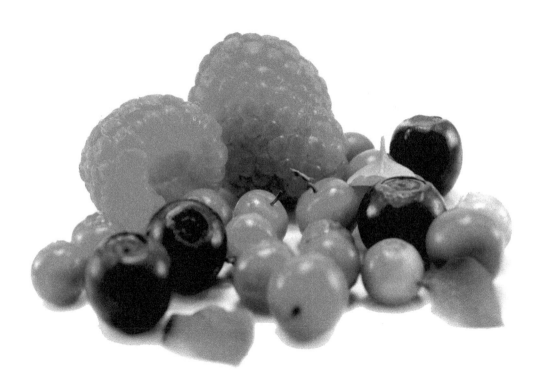

Chapter Eight

Self-Trust

Self-trust is the essence of heroism.
—Ralph Waldo Emerson

I had been learning how to move the frenetic energy in my body-mind, a reflection of the cultural chaos in the hectic world, to the heart. To soften rather than try harder. To choose real feelings. To choose real whole food. To choose real whole recovery.

For years I kept my big fat food frenzy secret from my family of origin. I yearned to come clean with them, but I could not. As if I would send it to them, I wrote this poem:

SECRETS
I don't want you to know
my secrets
and I'm dying to tell you.
If I keep them to myself,
clench them tight,
maybe they're not true,
maybe my clandestine rituals
are only imaginary friends,
and what I am doing is not really happening.

My heart,
at the end of my left arm,
curls in on itself.

> What lies behind us and what lies before us are tiny matters, compared to what lies within us.
> R. W. Emerson

85

Someday I will open my palm
and heart to you
and show you my truth.
Will you hold it tenderly?
Can you take good care of it?
I don't know now.
So I close my fist again.

Heartfulness is not about
brownies, whether we eat
them or not; it is about
how, why, when, and with
what mind and heart we
make our choices.

I couldn't send it, or maybe wouldn't. I had, by this time, stopped harming myself. I had begun to choose less and less harmful foods. Not perfect. I reduced the harm in brownies by making recipes from books listed in the bibliography. Or I ate them less often, or I ate only a few bites. My body was happier and I was leaning into health in the right direction. Heartfulness is not about brownies, whether we eat them or not; it is about how, why, when, and with what mind and heart we make our choices.

Eventually, even if we are terrified to break the silence, our burden gets too heavy to carry alone. One day, since we are social animals, we must share our despair, step out of our secrets.

How would I tell them? From Maine, where I lived, I wanted to send a note like this to them in Florida, where they wintered:

I am changing,
Mom and Dad,
I am changing.
I have found home in the heart,
I am learning to grow
in love
for myself
for my uniqueness,
whoever I am.
You do not fully know me.
I do not know myself,
I can't tell you who I am right now.

I am changing,

And I am heading to my own true home.

I could not send the poem. I wrote something more straightforward:

Dear Mom and Dad,

I am better now. But I want you to know that I have been struggling with food issues for years. Bulimia. Compulsive eating. Being too fat and being too thin. I have had individual therapy, and group work. They helped.

I love you both. This has nothing to do with you. I am eating differently from you now. I choose real foods, actual grow-from-the-ground foods that do not trigger me into eating frenzies. I am eating what helps me to feel the best and most centered. I am eating a whole foods, plant-based diet.

We can talk more about this if you want. Again, I am getting better and I love you. Love, Sue

This was the best I could do.

As I began to tell my story to family to friends, to support group peers, to therapists, to dieticians, there were many responses, some like sunlight inviting the new healthy sprouts in me to grow, others like a downpour, smashing the shoot back underground or into the mud:

"Oh, Susan, how could you do such a disgusting thing? That's gross. We saw a TV special last week on eating disorders. A young girl, who used those same words—food frenzy—sat on the floor all alone in the middle of the kitchen with open boxes of Fritos, Cheetos, Fig Newtons, Ritz crackers and Chunky Monkey Ben & Jerry's. There were wrappers, boxes and bags of junk strewn all over the floor. She ended up almost comatose. You don't do that, do you? That's really sick."

> If a story is in you it has got to come out.
> William Faulkner

"Well, we're really glad you are getting better and you got the help you need. We love you no matter what and we're proud of all you've done."

"Good thing you weren't anorexic. That would have been scary and awful."

"I never would have known. You look so 'together.' I always thought you were perfect."

"I guess you've really been through a lot. I thought I was the only one messed up in this group."

"I always figured you were bulimic."

"I eat so much at times that I have always wished I could throw it all up, but I just can't make myself do that. I'm kind of jealous."

"Oh, so that's how you stay so thin. Maybe I'll try it."

"Sounds like you've been on a long journey of your own and never left Maine."

"You're eating only whole plant foods? That sounds crazy."

"I hope you won't turn into one of those vegan freaks. "

Some wanted to fix me. Some never mentioned it again. Some badgered and nagged. Some pretended they never knew. If I were to do it again, I would have asked myself some important questions before disclosing the undisclosed, before opening what I had held so tight all those years:

How does this person I am thinking about telling handle pain and suffering in his or her own life?

Has this person taken a deep look at his or her own struggles?

Does this person open or shut down in adversity?

What is the state of this person's heart?

What does my intuition say—that part of me that is not the same as reason, that cannot talk the language of the head—what is my heart telling me?

Will this person's unwholesome relationship to toxic foods keep them closed to the latest nutritional findings?

Can this person listen without judgment or will this person jump in, change the subject, crack a joke, or interrupt?

We all have huge history living in us—past beliefs, old wounds, painful memories, other people's voices dancing in our heads. Many characters play in us. Each inner sub-personality has its own voice and needs to be heard to free us to hear a larger more heartful view.

When should we tell? After we come out to ourselves. After we heal from perfectionism. When we start listening to our own voice.

What should we tell? What the heart wants heard. What feels safe. Our felt experience. Our feelings.

> You gain strength, courage and confidence by every experience in which you really stop to look fear in the face.
>
> Eleanor Roosevelt

How should we tell? By being present, conscious of our own motivations and intentions for telling. With great spaciousness and compassion for ourselves and for the listener, who may find it excruciatingly difficult to hear what we have to say; all the time, staying in alignment with our heart and the truth of how things are, the truth of what real nutrition is for the body, the truth of what's best for the planet, the truth of what we have experienced and learned.

Who should we tell? First tell yourself; really, really get honest with yourself. Really, really own all those voices inside creating that great force which wants to take you over. Write. Draw. Listen, in your coming out to yourself, for a voice that is bigger than food frenzy. Listen for a wiser voice. You will come to clarity.

And where? At the heart. In the heart. From the heart.

Antidotes to Food Frenzy

Find Your Heart (Eight minutes)

If you have been practicing finding the heart, feeling into the heart, staying in the heart as much as you can, returning to the heart as soon as you can, then you may have begun to see that the deep heart is hugely spacious. When we sit in the heart center, there is room for all we bring to it. Meditation teacher Stephen Levine says, "Make space in your heart for your pain and make space in your pain for your heart." Whatever causes you pain in your life, bring it to the heart. The heart knows what to do with our suffering. Inside the pain, see if you can open your heart to it, not judge it or yourself. When you can and if you do, you will know how and when and with whom to talk about food frenzy. Give

> To know what you prefer instead of humbly saying Amen to what the world tells you you ought to prefer, is to have kept your soul alive.
>
> R. L. Stevenson

yourself fresh air. Beauty. Space. Warm comforters. Hugs.

You'll notice over time that the body loves real wholesome plant-based food, good rest, appropriate movement, kind human touch, deep easy breaths, and good clean water. Our true body does not crave junk. The heart needs our own love, attention and true nourishment from both real plant foods and lots of non-food sources.

For eight minutes right now, (practice is more important than reading the next chapter) practice the discipline of sitting in your heart and feeling the heart. Simple; not always easy, but avoiding the discipline of heartfulness practices will not fix food frenzy. You have learned many practice-based skills: tennis, golf, playing piano, brushing and flossing your teeth, changing a baby's diaper, painting. Whatever. Now learn to support your heart.

For eight minutes, you can use these words as you find refuge in the heart (adapted from the compassionate practices of Vietnamese mindfulness teacher Thich Nhat Hahn): Breathing in, I rest in the heart. Breathing out, I smile.

Stay right here, right now, in these moments. If your mind pulls you into the past or future, come back again and again and yet again to your center, to your core, which is always in this present moment.

Repeat, with each inhale and each exhale for eight minutes: Breathing in, I rest in the heart. Breathing out, I smile. Rest. Smile.

Notice how the repetition of the words returns you to center, and how the returning to your heart increases awareness and brings you home again and again.

Know Thyself

When you are ready to accept your heart, your values, your struggles, your hopes for your own future, then what can you say about your new way of eating? If and when it feels right, how can you claim the new part of yourself to others? When you go out to eat, can you say out loud, "I no longer eat meat?" Or, "I don't eat processed food?" or "I only eat dessert once a week. Thank you." What are the changes you've made to help your body be happier? What are your values around food? Can you say them out loud? Can you step into them? Own them? Eventually those around you come to know and accept "this is the way you eat," as long as you are very clear that "this is the way I eat." Can you state their importance to you and your physical, mental and emotional health, regardless of what others believe or do or say?

Sit now and write what you would tell, what needs to be spoken, your fears, your mess-ups, your anger, your journey, your triumphs. Write what you want loved ones or trusted ones to know. What do you do with food? What is so bad? What is so scary? Speak it or parts of it out loud to yourself. Then (you'll know the right time) speak it or parts of it to a trusted other. Begin the process of telling your secrets so they do not fester within nor get passed on (as family secrets do) to the next generation. Then notice how your body feels. Lighter? Less burdened? Relieved? Better? Worse? Simply notice and let yourself feel whatever you feel. Notice if you judge yourself, the very act you do not want anyone else to do. Write it all. Remember self-compassion.

Get Real with Food

Claim your truth and acknowledge your worth. The first coming out is to yourself. It is as much energetic as verbal, maybe even pre-verbal, a feeling: This is how I feel when I eat that way. And THIS is how I feel when I eat that way. It is at first a whispering, a knowing, an internal awareness. Have you admitted your suffering? Do you acknowledge your struggles? And what about your triumphs (how's that list coming along?)? To speak the truth to others comes only after we know our truth, and we begin to live it. It might be enough for while to say, "No, thank you, that pie looks delicious but I am not hungry right now." Or, "thanks anyway, I am really enjoying these vegetables from the garden." Do it. Maybe it's enough to do what your body loves, to do it more and more often, to feel the benefits, to be feeling comfortable, to dwell in heartfulness before you come out to others.

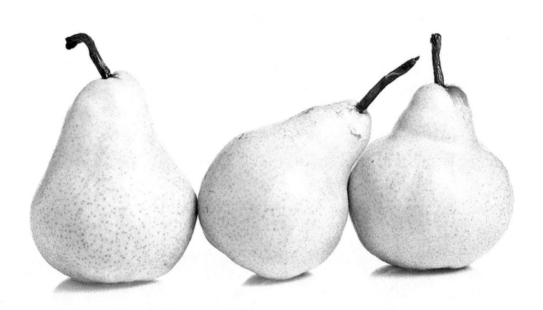

Chapter Nine

Facing The Dragon

To change a person must face the dragon of his appetite with another dragon, the life energy of the soul.

—Rumi

Like a corkscrew,
recovery bores its way
in.
Deeper,
cleaner,
clearer,
the twists of the heart
reveal the
sludge.
The turns of the
whole
purify particles.

While the arms
lift
upward
toward something
Greater,
the
probe
spirals

The road to breaking free from the dragon of appetite is not a path of perfection. It is a path of practice.

downward,

anticipating,

anticipating,

just that moment

when

poof,

the precious

wine

can breathe,

and what's in the

bottle

opens.

—Susan Lebel Young

Like the gifts in the wine waiting to be uncorked, health, wholeness, holiness, are inside us all along. Health, wholeness and holiness are never missing. They are not "other." They have, perhaps, in our repeated food frenzies, become buried beneath the fake foods we stuffed into our physical body while neglecting our famished spirit. Because the body will move toward wholeness, health is present in us, waiting for us to allow it to flourish. Practice calling forth the life energy of the soul will lead to self-trust and self-care. It's no accident that whole, real, natural, plant foods lead to whole body, mind and spiritual heatlh. Attention to wholeness in nutrition, in self-care and self-trust underlie freedom from food frenzy.

The road to breaking free from the dragon of appetite is not a path of perfection. It is a path of practice. Why? Because food frenzy is a persistent dragon. Because we must match the energy of what troubles us and the energy of a huge market economy which would have us buy and consume fake processed products loaded with addictive fats, sugars and salt. We must match the outer cultural pulls with equal or greater inner vigor in order to know internal peace. This dragon of appetite convinces us that—right now—

we need this new bottle of supplements, even though what we bought last week remains unopened. Chromium. Holy Basil. Green powders. Protein bars. When overwhelmed with TV ads, road signs, blinking neon, magazine full-page spreads, we often disassociate from our center. We leave ourselves and we leave what the heart knows about real nutrition. How else could I, could any of us whom this dragon invades, run from store to store buying Little Debbie cakes and eating much of our stash of high-fat high-sugar, sweet, high-calorie food while driving the car, convinced that we cannot stop, hating ourselves later, and then re-entering the world to function highly, as most of us do?

Food frenzy has a life and energy of its own. Food frenzy is not so much about devouring food as being devoured by it. Snack Attacks and Cookie Monsters are not the same as loving to eat. Junk is not love.

> We must match the outer cultural pulls with equal or greater inner vigor in order to know internal peace.

The Dragons of Appetite

I am forty.

It is January 1989. Today the temperature in Portland, Maine, is 10 degrees. Blowing and blustery, with the wind chill factor, it feels 15 below zero. Returning home from volunteering in Alisa's third-grade classroom, only two blocks away, I slam the back door to keep the outside freeze from taking over the kitchen. I put the little package I am carrying on the counter. I brought home this gift from the classroom "for the family." They would love some homemade desserts, I have convinced myself. Truth is, I am the only one in the house who will eat broken and smashed cookies. I helped with a baking project this morning, an innovative lesson Mrs. Neilsen created to encourage her very active third-graders to expand their knowledge of multiplication and to begin to learn fractions. "If we double this recipe, how much flour will we need? If we cut it in half, how much sugar goes in the bowl? What is one third of a tablespoon?"

Filled with the resulting freshly-baked chocolate chip cookies, the small brown paper bag radiates warmth. I have already licked fingers full of batter and shared liberally in the finished product with the school children. I am not hungry. In fact I am almost ill. I am full, sickened with that dull ache and sour feeling in the belly from inhaling buttery, sugary confection. No matter. I want more. The dragon screams, "Now!"

The cookie remains are warm. I see melted bits of chocolate now, seeping through the outside of the brown paper bag. Their aroma comes with them. I am freezing. They could give me a lift, I reason. If I were more alert, I would hear this as the beginning of the dragon's seduction. Two hours with thirty or so wound-up nine-year-olds has drained my energy. I tighten against the frigid elements shivering with my shoulders stiff around my ears. In this vulnerable moment, I am perfect prey.

> Nothing great was ever achieved without enthusiasm.
> R. W. Emerson

The smell of melted brown sugar, butter and chocolate triggers the dragon, "A little something could help you relax, make you feel better. Just one won't hurt." But I have already had many, maybe ten—most likely more, who's counting?—and polishing off the bag will not fix anything. I am about to succumb to the dragon's appetite. I have forgotten that all cravings eventually pass. I have forgotten who I am and what my heart really wants.

In these moments of forgetting, the room loses all its detail, fades into a background blur. Nothing exists but my drive for the cookies. I gotta have 'em. My head spins, eyes fixed, glazed. I am no longer present. Numb to everything else, I am dazed and hyper-focused. Human ego strength alone is not enough to halt this force.

In this moment, I need a way to call forth dormant parts of me, parts that are, until now, inaccessible. I need a practice of connecting to the deep inner heart and the life energy it gives. I need it now, grounded in my body, and available in this ever-present moment. The mind has not been helpful here; I need the strength of the heart.

In the movie *The Horse Whisperer*, Robert Redford plays the part of a man confronted with a traumatized horse. Redford's character must use his skills to "listen" to the horse's subtle messages to heal the anger, fear and self-protection, and to calm the animal's acting out. He waited for the horse to trust again. He forced nothing. He honored the way of the horse and held in his mind and heart the innate goodness of that wounded being, as difficult and challenging as the horse behaved. When I watched this movie, I saw myself and my clients in that horse, saw Redford as the therapist. He did not lecture or punish rebellious behavior. What did he do? He gave space. When we are hurting, we need openness.

I am forty-one.

Spring, 1990. I am at the dinner table with Alisa and Zac. She sits, her two upper front teeth protruding beyond her narrow lip, waiting for braces next week. Her smile—big, ear-to-ear—is the smile of a ten-year-old. Her straight shoulder-length black hair falls into her homemade organic applesauce, bangs drooping in her face. She can reach her hair with her tongue, and loves to catch one single strand as she mixes it with her mashed potatoes. She wears a pastel pink grosgrain ribbon behind her ears, but it is so thin it does not hold back her hair. Her green Icelandic sweater shows a few peanut butter stains from her school lunch.

> People become really quite remarkable when they start thinking that they can do things. When they believe in themselves they have the first secret of success.
>
> Norman V. Peale:

Zac, age eight, shifts from side to side in his ladder-backed chair, rocking it until it topples over. As he falls, he takes out his napkin, which trips the plastic kiddy-fork, which lands on his tender ear. He bleeds. Pouting, he gets up, we settle him, and he jumps up to go the refrigerator to get more orange juice. He drops the blue and white-checkered pitcher and covers the oak floor. I am too tired to mop it up right now, so I leave it, heart racing, blood boiling. Sitting again, he faces the big red clock on the wall, although he does not read the time. But I do, and I wish the time were different. I wish dinner were over. I wish I could be out with my friends. I wish. I wish…

On each salad-size plate, I place some lentils, covered with a dollop of Heinz ketchup—for Zac it has to be Heinz or he'll throw a tantrum, not unlike Redford's horse. Each plate also gets a few green peas, which I know neither will eat, and mashed potatoes. Chunky mashed potatoes with the red skins left on—this they like.

Zac spills his milk. Alisa rolls her eyes. Zac catches the gesture and cries. "She is always teasing me, Mom. I can't stand it when she does that."

She yells back.

I wish I had a Horse Whisperer here to calm these wild animals. I yearn to skip dinner altogether and go straight to Dunkin' Donuts down the road. Chocolate-glazed, cream filled.

I churn. I want to eat. No, I want to stuff. I want to get my children to bed and eat the whole box of Wheat Thins my husband bought for himself. I want to wait until they are asleep and eat all the peanut butter Nabs I bought for their lunches this week. I want to be alone and devour the Nutter Butter Peanut Butter Sandwich Cookies I have tucked away.

But I hear the life energy of the soul in me. It is demanding drastic action. "Get these kids outside," it commands, "let them duke it out. Let them throw food. Join them."

"What?" I question these marching orders.

"Get outside NOW."

> Do one thing every day that scares you.
> Eleanor Roosevelt

Something in me accepts the battle cry. I believe its soulfulness.

"Let's go," I say to both bewildered kids. Their mouths hang open. Their eyes lock—allies all of a sudden.

"What?"

"We're going to have a food fight."

I hear myself mouth these words, as much surprised by them as my children. I have never had a food fight, never been allowed. Not ladylike enough. A bit too out of control.

They do not believe me. "Ma, what are you, crazy?"

"Now. Out. Let's go. C'mon."

With wide-opened eyes, Zac smooshes his little fingers in the applesauce, dragging a trail of it across the already soaked floorboards, running out the door, letting it slam behind his back in Alisa's face. Laughing, Alisa makes fists and pushes mashed potatoes into them and then out, and a bit through, the screen door. I take Jell-o.

> Freedom is the spaciousness provided by the whisperings of the heart.

Once we hit the back yard, we make a big fracas, a melee of hands in faces, backs to tummies, food squished everywhere. Jell-o colors hair. Applesauce smears shirts. Mashed potato gobs in the head. Grass stains add to the mix. Dinner fertilizes the ground.

We go at it until we can't anymore, until we roll on the ground. We are exhausted, and released.

Alisa laughs; Zac stands up strong.

I cry because I have said, "NO," to the incipient pent-up binge, "No."

"NO," I say this time to the appetite which would normally have me dutifully stay in that chaotic kitchen, clean up oh-so-neatly, put them to bed, and then attack the cupboards and fridge.

Big tears. I have never felt so free with food. With a food fight, I have stopped the war in my head. With the life energy of the soul, I have faced the dragon.

Antidotes to Food Frenzy

Find Your Heart (Nine minutes)

The irony of the title *Food Fix* is that we may not need fixing. When we drop into the heart, when we enlist the energy of the soul, we see our struggles in a new light and new ideas come to us. Food fights are not the answer here. Freedom is the spaciousness provided by the whisperings of the heart. If we look the dragon right in the eye, we will see that it will not eat us. Yet we will not be able to face the dragon at the moment it strikes unless we have practiced over and over again.

Feel into the center of your chest.

> You yourself, as much as anybody in the entire universe, deserve your love and affection.
>
> Buddha

Stay.

Let your feet relax.

Let your arms be loose and heavy.

Let your breath be full as it moves in three dimensions around your heart.

Let the eyes release and relax.

Let the brain float free and loose in the skull.

Let the shoulders drop away from the ears.

Let the legs be heavy.

Let the tongue be loose and heavy.

Unclench the jaw.

Now that you have let go of holding in the whole body, let your attention rest in the heart.

Let the center of your chest light up your awareness.

For nine minutes, let the heart be foreground in your mind.

You are practicing for when you need to recognize the dragon and want to refrain from letting it win, when you need to relax into the heart and repeat it again and again and again until the dragon gets the message.

Right now, for nine minutes, and then as often as possible, breathe into the heart. Rest in the heart for nine minutes. Feel what it feels like and how it is different from screaming cravings and rushing thoughts in the head.

Know Thyself

We are now about halfway through this book. As you may have noticed, this book is not a book of scientific or psychological information. It is a book of practice. A book for action through skill-building. If you only read, nothing changes. And if nothing changes, nothing changes in the body/mind complex or in our behaviors. Insights do not create change. "Oh, this is interesting stuff" will not calm the food frenzy. We need to meet that dragon with our whole being. We come home to the heart to heal. We return, and re-tune to the heart over and over again, moment-to-moment, day after day. The calm heart comes

between you and chaotic food frenzy. Low-fat whole foods plant-based eating is not a new diet. It is a new lifestyle. It is finally letting the body learn to truly love what it naturally loves.

Write or draw the dragon. What are you up against? Is it a person, is it a monster, a fiery furnace, a tornado, a mean coach, rebellious teenager, tantrum-throwing toddler? Know it. Feel it. Capture its energy. Write it. Draw it.

Get Real with Food

Try new foods. Go to the grocery store, farmer's market, produce stand or other local marketplace. Walk around. Look at the colors, shapes, textures of the produce. Find something that you have never tasted. Buy it, bring it home. What will you do with it? Get creative. Will you eat it raw, cook it, throw it into a salad or soup? Be playful. Have fun.

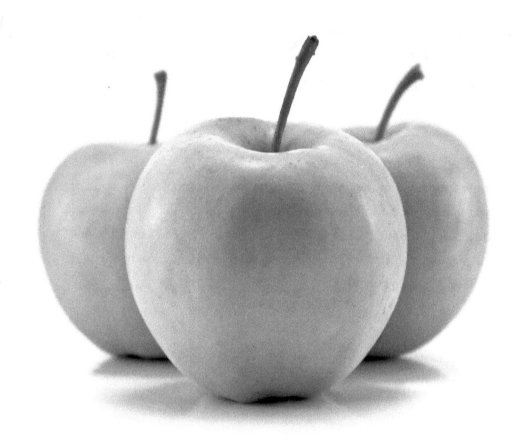

Chapter Ten

Enough

"I am not enough."
There is not enough
chocolate in the world to
gobble up such
mental junk food. And yet I
chew and chew on this
mind's garbage.

I am not thin enough.
I am not smart enough.
I am not tall enough.
Blonde enough, fit enough....

—Susan Lebel Young

I am enough, the heart repeats. "This moment is enough," my mindfulness teachers tell me. "You're fit enough," the trainer affirms. "You're thin enough," my doctor reminds me. "You're smart enough," my students show me. "You're compassionate enough," my children say. "You listen enough" my clients seem to think. "You know enough," my husband insists. Yet there are louder voices in my head, familiar negativity screaming just the opposite, spewing out the declarations of the critic, the judge. "You are not good enough. You will never be good enough. Not thin enough. Not strong enough. Not smart enough. Not pretty enough."

I have learned to recognize these old familiar warning signals which would trigger unhealthy behaviors. As I detach from their impact, I go back in my mind. I search my childhood. How old are these messages? Whose voices are they? Where do they originate? Even as I inquire, I am back in Catholic school, afraid of being scolded:

1959. I am ten years old at St. Joseph's Academy for girls, where we memorize the blue paperback Baltimore Catechism:

Who made you?

God made me.

Why did God make you?

God made me to show His goodness and to make me happy with Him in Heaven.

By mandate, on Saturdays we go to confession at St. Joseph's Church, a huge Gothic cathedral, empty except for the deep echoing whispers of an unseen man behind a dark screen in the confessional.

"Forgive me Father for I have sinned. It has been one week since my last confession."

I list everything I remember that I have done "wrong" since last Saturday. Always worrying whether he can identify me by my blonde hair shining through the separating screen or by my short stature, I disguise my voice. I know I have to tell my transgressions to Father Murphy and God the Father in order to get to Heaven someday. But I do not want anyone telling my parents.

During my early religious training, we have many opportunities to sin from week to week because thoughts, words, feelings and deeds all qualify. I am a good kid, really. The oldest of seven, I am Mother's little helper, the one who remembers and assists all the others in signing birthday cards for Mom and Dad. I rock babies daily, do chores, get up early to help in the kitchen. On Saturday mornings at eleven o'clock, though, I dig deep to castigate myself. I have been born with original sin, which means I am inherently flawed, have a tendency to be bad, and need to do what some holy male authority orders to atone for it. But I can never erase it. As I understand it, only men can do this for me—the priests, or Christ, or God the Father. Even then, at least in my girlhood mind, original sin isn't gone. In my bones, I have internalized that I must be vigilant as I live with this wrongdoing of Eve's—a woman—and as I carry this badness in the world.

"Thursday I didn't have enough money for candy, so I stole a quarter from my Father's dresser…during math class, I wasn't interested enough, so I shot a rubber elastic band into Mrs. Schmidt's frizzy gray hair…this morning I wasn't honest enough because I stole again: I ate the whole head of a chocolate bunny that really belonged to my brother, Mike… I lied to my mother; I didn't clean well enough because I didn't vacuum under my bed."

I wish I could confess the way my grandfather tells us he does, "Hi. It's Gus Albert. Same as last week."

But I'm not old enough or cute enough or funny enough to pull that off.

"For your penance say five 'Our Fathers and three 'Hail Marys."

"Thank you, Father."

I do not feel purer or lighter after these weekly ritualistic cleansings. Guilty is what I feel. Not holy enough is what I feel, for maybe forgetting something or—worse yet—for leaving something out on purpose. Never do I dare to tell Father Murphy that Maureen and I have an afternoon club in her basement from which we exclude other girls. Or that, walking home from St. Joseph's Academy to the club meetings, we skip down Stephen's Avenue on purpose to wait for public school boys just dismissed from Longfellow School. Or that the point of the two-member club is to find and draw "dirty pictures." Even with all the penance-prayers I dutifully perform, I do not expect them to be enough to save my soul. I expect to go to hell for sure.

So when the principal, Sister Adelina, asks me to lead a decade of the Rosary at a Mass for Mary, during May, Mary's month, I am excited. It means that Father Murphy doesn't know me from the confessional, and that he never told

Mrs. Schmidt about my elastic-shooting. It also means I have a chance to redeem myself. Maybe I am smart enough or dependable enough to heal my original badness with good works in the world, like Christ.

You see, in fifth grade, I am always being caught doing something "wrong." My navy blue jumper and brown oxford shoes arrived in late August, the only parochial school uniform whose white polyester blouse had short sleeves. "Miss Lebel," Sister Adelina admonished, "These sleeves are not long enough. They must cover your wrists. You should be ashamed of yourself."

I was. This incident caused a very controversial discussion about whether or not it is appropriate to attend a Catholic girls' elementary school exposing my ten-year-old elbows.

Lively and spirited, I am also not quiet enough. I talk and laugh more than the Sisters of Mercy want.

Two days a week, four-feet tall Sister Eucharia bounces into our small classroom to teach French. So tiny that her habit does not fit, she constantly adjusts her white starched headpiece, which slips all around her head. Clucking her tongue against the roof of her mouth, she has trouble keeping her complete set of upper and lower dentures in place. With her squeaky voice and her animated body, she darts around the classroom, waving her long wooden rubber-tipped pointer in the air. All year, we work to memorize "The Ant and the Grasshopper, La Cigale et la Fourni:"

> La Cigale, ayant chanté
>
> Tout l'été,
>
> Se trouva fort dépourvue
>
> Quand la bise fut venue:…something like that.

At least once in every class, her top denture loosens. Using her tongue to pull it back onto her upper ridge, she makes a loud juicy, sloppy, end eventually slappy sound. Then she picks right up as if nothing had happened, "La Cigale et la Fourni."

With the falling habit, the miniature bouncing body, the flapping teeth, the loud slurp, I erupt in silliness. Under my breath, behind my cupped hands holding back sound, I stifle a chortle. I cannot look at Maureen, Nancy or Michelle because I know they are all giggling, too, and we can be in big trouble for laughing. Being happy is not part of my parochial education.

Because I "cannot meet behavior expectations in class," and because of my elbows, I suppose, I get a "D" in deportment. I am a straight "A" student with a "D" in Deportment. I believe I am not good enough.

So I am eager to lead the Rosary. I even know the Hail Mary prayer, which makes up the Rosary, in French. But today I get to say the first half out loud all by myself in English. Everyone else will respond together with the second half. Ten times. I feel important.

I have known the Hail Mary by heart for years. My great-aunt is a nun, my great-uncle a priest. By the age of ten, I have received a gift set or two of my own Rosary beads. As a maturing young girl, whenever I ask my mother questions about menstrual periods, she answers, among other helpful responses, "Pray to the Blessed Virgin Mary."

Wondering how that would help, and what a blessed virgin might know about budding sexuality, I nevertheless pray the Rosary often:

> *Hail Mary full of grace,*
> *The Lord is with Thee,*
> *Blessed art Thou among women*
> *And blessed is the fruit of thy womb, Jesus*
>
> *Holy Mary, Mother of God*
> *Pray for us sinners now*
> *And at the hour of our death*
> *Amen.*

All the girls from the fifth, sixth, seventh and eighth grades walk silently from the first floor classrooms to the small musty chapel on the second floor.

Ceremoniously, we dip our little-girl fingers into the holy water font at the entrance, and one by one, bless ourselves with the sign of the Cross, wet hands to the forehead first.

"In the name of the Father, and of the Son, and of the Holy Ghost. Amen."

My gut stirs. I feel honored. I can't wait for my turn. Now it is here, and I have every intention to pray to Mary in earnest. I have a special relationship with Mary. She is woman, and I sense she loves me, which I'm not so sure about God, the Father and the Son. Proudly, I begin:

"Hail Mary, Mother of God, pray for us sinners now and at the hour of our death. Amen."

Silence.

Immediately, I know it is wrong. I know I am wrong. I have not done this well enough. I had skipped all the way to "Amen." I had left no opening for anyone to respond. Frozen, I have no idea how to recover or what to do next.

With all of the fifth, sixth, seventh, eighth grade girls, and Father Murphy present, Sister Mary Frances barks firmly and caustically, "Miss Lebel, next time you expect to lead the Rosary, you'd better know the 'Hail Mary.' Miss Lebel, you should be ashamed of yourself."

I feel miniscule. As I curl in on myself, even at ten, I think, "If Mary is so full of grace, I wonder if she cares that I messed up her prayer?"

> To be yourself in a world that is constantly trying to make you something else is the greatest accomplishment.
> R. W. Emerson

I have great appreciation for the positive spiritual underpinnings of my religious upbringing. Roman Catholicism rooted me in a strong mystical core, crucial to my healing today, important in how I live and what I teach. I used to pretend I was St. Theresa, even wanted to change my name legally to Theresa. Really. Yet now as adult, I sit, wanting to know that I am enough, to feel that this moment is enough, and I re-experience the scars from the lack of kindheartedness, compassion and joy of several misguided authorities. I am working to have the heart embrace "enoughness," so that I no longer need to fill up with Mars bars and pints of cool creamy gooey milky treats. There isn't, there will never be, enough junk food to fill spiritual and emotional hungers.

> We must meet the force of great suffering with even greater compassion and love.

Enough. I am slowly coming to see that this breath, right here, right now, is nourishing; that this moment is filling; that this sitting here is nurturing; and that this heart is full. Yet sometimes, even though the actual shaming is far in the past, I feel myself disappointing Father Murphy, Sister Mary Frances and the whole middle school of St. Joseph's Academy all over again. The old, habitual message, reinforced weekly in confession, is embedded; "I am not enough."

Because of early "not enough" messages, we must be vigilant in the present, noticing the reprimands of the past arising again and again. The heart knows they are not true, but the old voices in the head may get more of our attention. What we pay attention to matters. We must meet the force of great suffering with even greater compassion and love.

Antidotes to Food Frenzy

Find Your Heart (Ten minutes)

For ten minutes, sit.

Sit now.

Stop.

Breathe into your core. Let this be your affirmation: I am enough. When we know we are enough, we no longer need to fill up on toxic food.

Know Thyself

Create a plan of eating for today and/or tomorrow. Write it down. What kind of whole plant-based meal will you have for breakfast? What about lunch and dinner? Think real, whole foods, not fractionated elements like carbs, fats and proteins. Think, "What five colorful veggies will I put in my salad? (Tonight I had purple cabbage, red pepper, green avocado, yellow summer squash and orange carrots). "What kind of green vegetable will I steam?" (Tonight I steamed Brussels sprouts). "What kind of fruit do I want as dessert or snack?" (Tonight I made a smoothie from frozen peaches, dates, unsweetened rice milk and golden flax seeds.) Go online for help, if you need ideas. See the bibliography at the end of this book for websites and books.

Write in your journal: I am enough. I am enough. I am enough. Keep it up. It is true. With practice, you will believe it.

Get Real with Food

Today, choose different colors, different textures. By now, with the practices of adding more and more real food, you may be beginning to experience that real, whole, plant-based food is enough. We come to crave healthy foods. Really. Transformation happens if we practice eating well. Really. Fresh fruit, vegetables, whole grains, legumes, raw nuts and seeds are enough because we are wired genetically to eat what comes from the earth, from gardens, from forests. One key to feeling "enough" is to practice getting enough variety, texture, color and enough volume from the antioxidants, phytochemicals, fiber and plant-derived nutrient diversity. Then our bodies will be satisfied and fulfilled.

> Nature is just enough; but men and women must comprehend and accept her suggestions.
> Antoinette B. Blackwell

Chapter Eleven

Enough Again

You never know what is enough until you know
what is more than enough.

—William Blake

What is "enough" in this culture? How do I learn enough when Barron's, the Dow Jones Business and Financial Weekly, reported in 1996 that, "the food giants spend close to $45 billion a year in advertising to encourage consumption." Yale psychologist Kelly Brownell calls the result a toxic environment. If we listen to what is being fed to us, we are in trouble.

Some of us are lured by "fat-free, sugar-free fruit-juice unsweetened cookies." Others are seduced by non-fat anything.

I am forty-six.

It's Friday. I finish a full day of counseling individuals, ending with the facilitation of an hour-and-a-half group. Clients discussed heavy issues today; fear of death; fear of not living wholeheartedly and fully; moves that leave behind friends, supportive family, secure jobs; awareness of how much energy it takes to confront the past and move on. I love being a counselor. This calling fills me in many ways. Yet in this moment I am emotionally drained, having worked to listen with empathic presence and unconditional positive regard all day.

I pack my book bag, my tea, my notes, and some paperwork to take home. "Good-bye," I say to the people in the office.

> When this moment is
> enough, life is enough.
> Stephen Levine

"Have a nice weekend."

I head out the door, walk from the building to my sedan. My mind runs wild with how much I have left to do later today: go home, call Jon, pick up the kids, get dinner, rush to teach a class at the university. My body revs with kinetic energy, too. Keep moving. Stay in motion. Do something, and whatever it is, it will never be enough. What is enough? What would be enough work? What would be enough activity? What would be good enough mothering?

The thinking mind stirs:

"Should I go straight home and start grazing through the kitchen? Or should I stop at the new organic bakery for a sample of their warm, freshly-baked peanut butter chocolate chip cookies? Or should I go to the super grocery store and grab a quick something? Or should I stop at the natural foods store and get some velvety non-dairy frozen dessert?"

All this mental energy swarms in my head which still spins from the group, reeling from a long day, revisiting the suffering of clients—clients who have hours ago gone home—and at the same time rehearsing the presentation due later at the university. "Am I prepared enough? Have I read enough? Will it be good enough?"

The chatter quickens my body-mind. Push on. Adrenaline rush, heart pounding. In a driven panic, I hurry, scurry to the Mom and Pop corner store. Furtively, I buy a pint of Ben & Jerry's chocolate chip cookie dough ice cream. So no one will know, I place it in the cup holder between the driver's seat and the passenger's side. I scoop fingerfuls as I drive until some of it melts. Then I peel the paper from the edges and lick the soft melted part, tongue making circles as it follows the creamiest parts. Ahhh.

How do we learn "enough" in a world where our bingeing is the goal of the grocery industry? How do we learn "enough" when addictive food-like substances are pushed, legally, easily, cheaply, as if to answer all our ills? How do we learn "enough" when advertisements for laxative preparations, antacid tablets, and diuretic teas promise to take care of the excess? Is this not socially-acceptable purging? How do we learn "enough," when over-the-counter drugs tout a cure for the disease of acid reflux? Acid reflux is not a disease. Rather it is a symptom of over-consumption caused by burger/fries/milk shake ads in the first place. How do we learn "enough?"

Stopping daily on the way home from work for a little something entrenches old patterns. Yet over time, with heart practices as an antidote, something shifts. Even when we eat what we wish we hadn't, even when we disappoint ourselves, it matters what we do next.

This Friday I become conscious after the numbing out. Awareness comes to me. I wake up. This day, even after I scarf down a pint, I return my attention to the big heart in the center of my chest front and back. I listen. From just between the shoulder blades, I hear, "Rest now, shhhh."

> Leaning into the deep heart for support does not take extra time. It takes a shift in attention.

Leaning into the deep heart for support does not take extra time. It takes a shift in attention. Our tendency is to want to figure out the "ice cream thing," to fight with it, to throw the pint away, or to eat it all now. Push, pull. Eat it; don't eat it. Hide it; throw it out. When we listen to the heart, though, we know the truth of Einstein's words—that we cannot solve a problem with the same mind, the same consciousness, which created the problem in the first place.

> Stopping, putting heart space between food fix ideas and actual food frenzy is perhaps the biggest message in this book.

Nevertheless, many of us often resist stopping. Stopping, putting heart space between food fix ideas and actual food frenzy is perhaps the biggest message in this book. We all, by nature it seems, fight against what we know is needed; a sacred pause, a dropping into the heart. So after eating, I turn my attention to a warmer, more welcoming place. What I do after a binge is crucial. What we do after a binge, how we live moment-to-moment, can begin a profound change.

Antidotes to Food Frenzy

Find Your Heart (Eleven minutes)

In the middle of any food frenzy, the heart waits, sometimes in the car, sometimes in a rocking chair, sometimes on the meditation cushion, or the yoga mat, or a computer desk. We never know in advance what the heart will tell us, what the heart will show us. When we live inside our center, we find peace. When we live outside our own center, we suffer.

Consider a way to intervene before a binge. The pause between thoughts such as, I-want-it-and-I-want-it-now, allows us to shift our attention from foods and behaviors that don't support us to habits that do. The more we practice, the better we get at waiting, at patience, at pausing when impulse arises. As we restrain ourselves, our thoughts/feelings might still be in frenzy. I want, gimme, I need. But we can choose to put off eating. In this eleven-minute Food-Fix-On-Hold, we can do what needs doing while the craving does what it will most likely do—come and go. We can walk, or take a bath, or return a phone call, or read, or write in our journal, or remind ourselves why we are making these changes, or simply practice dropping into the heart.

We can feel the fear, the anger, shame, whatever, putting food fix on hold as we do what needs doing in our Food-Fix-Gap. In this pause, ask if you are

> In the middle of any food frenzy, the heart waits.

really physically hungry. If not, what do you really need? If you are physically hungry, see what happens if you wait to feed yourself. Have some water. Make a cup of tea. (We can live a lot longer without food than without water.) Consciously decide what you truly want, rather than grab what is there. In the Food-Fix-On-Hold moments, ask what would truly nourish. If you get an answer like, "a Milky Way bar," stop again, pause again, drop into the heart and ask, "really?"

We can't control when we get hit with food images or bingeing thoughts. We do have choice about our behavior. We can control whether or not we pick up that Lorna Doone cookie or lick our tongues around an ice cream cone. We may indeed salivate when we notice that it's noon; but instead of heading to the refrigerator today, try a food-fix-on-hold for eleven minutes and see what happens.

Really notice. You may have thoughts like, "if I don't eat right now, I'll die. I won't survive. I'll starve to death. I'll wither away. If I don't have this ice cream sandwich this instant, I'll binge later." The mind can be shameless and crazy-making. Notice it all and go on hold for eleven minutes.

Today, begin to practice an eleven minute Food-Frenzy-Pause, a way to stop between the first sign of craving and diving in.

Know Thyself

Write in your journal. For eleven minutes, write what a binge is for you. Webster's defines "binge" as "riotous indulgence." What do you call a binge? Is it certain foods? In certain quantities? Or is it qualitative—adrenaline-rushed eating, or a sense of lack of control? Is it quantitative? Does a binge last over a discrete amount of time for you? Minutes? Hours? Days? What do you mean when you say you binge?

Write about how you find your way back to your heart after you disappoint yourself. When the pull of addictive fats, sugars and salts tug at you, how do you get yourself to pick up a fruit or a vegetable again? Do you need more information? See bibliography at the end. Do you need more support? How will you find it? Do you need more motivation? What motivates you?

Any time, and especially after food frenzy has taken over, **make a list of the reasons you want this heartfulness for yourself.** Do it again and again and again. You will generate new reasons each time.

With an open heart, read it often.

> Every great mistake has a halfway moment, a split second when it can be recalled and perhaps remedied.
>
> Pearl S. Buck

Get Real with Food

Make a food plan for tomorrow. Tonight, before you go to bed, after your dinners most nights and especially after eating what does not serve you or

Do you have the patience to wait until your mud settles, and the water is clear? Can you remain unmoving until the right action arises by itself?

Lao-tzu

your heart, make a rough plan of the low-fat, high-fiber, whole foods, plant-based food you will prepare and eat tomorrow. It might look something like this:

Breakfast: oats, blueberries, walnuts, decaf green tea

Lunch: big colorful salad with brown rice and edamame; tahini dressing

Dinner: Veggie chili with lots of carrots, tomatoes, onions; steamed spinach and corn on the cob;

Snacks: fruit and/or veggies

When we have a plan, even a loose one, even if we don't stick with it exactly, we are more likely to be able to resist the urgency of food frenzy triggers. When we also practice Food-Fix-On-Hold, we are more likely to want our planned meals. With a plan, you can then check your cupboards for ingredients, make a grocery list. Be prepared. A plan adds simplicity, can cut down the distracting and conflicting pull of non-foods and is one way to meet the dragon of appetite.

Part Three

Staying Awake

To journey into this interior world within
Love must already be awakened
For love to awaken in us:
Let go.
Let be.
Be silent.
Be still in gentle peace...
Learn mindfulness.
　　　　—Saint Theresa of Avila

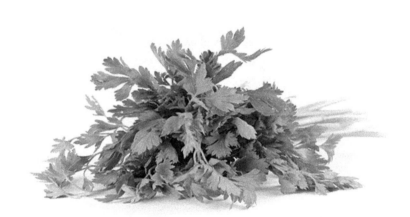

Chapter Twelve

Daily Heart Awakening

You have slept for millions and millions of years, why not wake up this morning?

—Kabir

I am fifty.

I am an adult, shopping at the Whole Grocer, and I have already grabbed a home-baked wheat-free-maple-syrup sweetened five-inch chocolate chip cookie. I eat it as I walk through produce, which I skip today on my way to the baked muffins. I can feel fear in me, my nervous system jacked up a notch, as I have once again broken a promise to myself. I am eating when I am not hungry and wolfing down junk. Jittery stomach, I am a failure again. I am in the book section and I spy a new hardcover which was not on the shelf last week. The title is seductive. Something about feeding myself in order to increase longevity. I browse through it. Hmm… Every single person who tries this program loses weight. Lots of weight. I am hooked. I buy the book and start the prescribed food plan.

But I cannot do this diet on my own, so I go to the website, call the author, sign up for a three–month specialty consultation service. I pay $1,300. With a vengeance, I absorb as much information as possible in a very short amount of time, start up with great energy. Surely this is it. Certainly this program, finally, will get me to a perfect lipid profile. Just a few days later, I decide this is not for me. Like dieting mentality, it does not feed my soul. Too restrictive. So I give it *up.*

Weeks later I read about an at-home program, spiritually based, for only five hundred dollars for the whole year. This is a bargain compared to the last scheme I bought. I watch the short video online. So many happy faces and before and after testimonials. I talk to convincing sales women on the phone. They have had my very same problems and this is the program that solved them. I jump in. Two days later, after I can no longer refuse the material which will arrive at my house every two weeks for the next year, I see that this plan will not nourish me deeply and I quit.

There is a special twelve-week "Blast-it-off" program at the gym. What a great idea. I will meet with a personal trainer twice a week, with a dietician once a week, I will wear a pedometer all day to see if I can take 10,000 steps, I will increase cardio workouts—all to reduce body fat, to lose weight, to increase fitness. There will be weigh-ins, body fat measuring and charts to keep. Lots of keeping score. All this for only nine hundred dollars. I sign up. Of course, without a way to discern in advance whether all this activity will feel right for me, will nurture me, I experience—one more time—the insight that this is not for me and I stop going to the gym.

> Peace and freedom come from seeing our inner light and from commitment to calming rituals which soothe the nervous system rather than agitate it, that settle the mind beyond impulsivity.

This restlessness is not the same as recovery from food frenzy. Short-term fixes are not like wrapping ourselves in the lasting cloak of ease and well-being. The question in recovery is not which is the next diet; rather, we ask ourselves: how can I come in close to my core before I make decisions? Peace and freedom come from seeing our inner light and from commitment to calming rituals which soothe the nervous system rather than agitate it, that settle the mind beyond impulsivity. Heartfulness is a discipline in which these daily rituals let us know we are already whole. We are enough. Whole, real food is enough. Paradoxically, there is nothing to fix. Without the practices of choosing wholeness, we forget and become fair game for the next attractive scheme.

To transform the energies of food frenzy, we practice time after time choosing real foods. We write our real story. We sit with the realness of our whole bodies and hearts. Wholesome rituals help us heal because they replace old harmful habits. Real plant food crowds out the junk food we used to choose. If we fill up on high-fiber fruits and vegetables, we are less likely to reach for empty calories. We feel a shift so that we less often choose chaos.

First, we come home to the heart as discipline; we need to remind ourselves to do it. We struggle, maybe for years, to find a home in the heart and in nutritious plant-based foods. Then we practice returning to the heart, as the old familiar habits and conditioning pull us away again and again. Eventually, there comes a time when living in the heart is a more natural way of being, becomes our home. Now practice does not take discipline. It is simply what we do. Eventually what we do is simple. We stop trying so hard, stop working so hard. We surrender into the heart, into life as it, just now, just here. And we notice, not by trying to change anything, not by any new diet, not by any rules, that the quality of our day and our food choices unfold with more peace.

> Eventually what we do is simple. We surrender into the heart, into life as it is, just now, just here.

Yet this dwelling in the heart must have anchors, tethers to help us stay, to remind us who we really are. It helps to begin the day waking up and asking for a change using the conscious rituals offered in this book rather than unconscious rituals of bingeing, or numbing out, or popping food in. With conscious rituals we set the tone for the waking hours. It used to be that every morning upon arising, I would trot to the bathroom, brush my teeth, and before sipping even a drop of water, I'd weigh myself then look in the mirror to see how fat my belly was. No matter what the measurements, I would pinch my skin in disgust. Every day, religiously you might say. We all have rituals. Others get up, read the paper, and have coffee to start the day; still others check the stock reports or their overnight e-mail. These are not wrong or bad; they may not, however, help us get conscious.

The mechanical god on the cold tile bathroom floor would display a number

It is a wholesome and necessary thing for us to turn again to the earth and in the contemplation of her beauties to know of wonder and humility.
Rachel Carson

to me, the weight that would determine how I felt all day. Daily, I performed this rite. If the numbers were up, anger, self-disgust, and depression would surface immediately. The obsession to diet drove me all day, determined to change this too-high number by tomorrow. My first acts of the day would then be to plan and write out what I would allow myself to eat; three meals, weighed and measured, nothing more.

Doing penance all day. If the numbers were down, the cold metal god granted permission to eat, to binge actually. I worshipped at the altar of that metal scale. Is that what the first commandment means by "Thou shalt not put false gods before me?" To weigh or not to weigh must be decided by each one of us. Is it a helpful ritual or does it take us out of our heart?

Clearly I needed a new way to wake up physically and metaphorically. In *Walden Pond*, Henry David Thoreau wrote, "Only the day dawns to which we are awake." He also wrote,

> Morning is when I awake and there is a dawn in me… We must learn to reawaken and keep ourselves awake, not by mechanical aids, but by an infinite expectation of the dawn… I know of no more encouraging fact than the unquestionable ability of man to elevate his life by conscious endeavor… To affect the quality of the day, that is the highest art.

Every morning now, if I remember to look when I first awaken, I see the paintbrush of the sunrise. Present, whether I am aware of it or not, are the first colors of the day. Oranges. Pinks. Often a mixture of orange and purple and yellow. Even on snowy or rainy days, out of that window I see the dark begin to brighten. I see night turn into day.

If I remember to look, I receive the pleasure of witnessing a miracle. If I acknowledge it, my day is already more abundant, even before I eat a morsel of food. There is magnificence in this early morning stillness. The colors of pre-dawn soon give way to the blue or gray of the unfolding sky. When I can remind myself to be attentive to it, I rest for a few conscious moments, aware of the privilege of making the acquaintance of the world again today. Twenty-four more hours. Something in me rises with the sun.

Rarely now, is my first morning thought, "I hate myself for eating crap last night." I need my morning rituals to help transform old automatic habits into true nourishment. The sun never hates itself. It does not appear today and chastise itself for not appearing yesterday or for last week's rain: "Oh, I really messed up yesterday. Look at all this mud and slush." The sun simply embraces the Earth again. We can learn from that.

> When people made up their minds that they wanted to be free and took action, then there was a change.
>
> Rosa Parks

Antidotes to Food Frenzy

Find Your Heart (Twelve minutes)

How you start the day sets the tone for the next many hours. What's in your heart as you get out of bed matters. Try a first-thing-in-the-morning ritual that makes sense to you. A heart-centered practice. Something simple. Something easy to remember, something you will love and look forward to doing. Gentle yoga. Or reading inspirational quotes. Or prayer. Or meditation. Or sitting and watching birds. Or slow mindful walking. Or writing in a journal a few pages every morning. Perhaps looking out the window and feeling blessed. Can you spend twelve minutes each morning, maybe even before you get out of bed, resting in your heart?

Try it now. Go lie down and imagine this is the first breath of the day. Feel it. Rest in the heart before you hit the ground running. Intend to come from the heart during the day. Twelve minutes. Now.

Know Thyself

Write out some of the rituals that have been so repetitive as part of food frenzy: cruising through drive-ins, bingeing alone in the car; choosing popcorn for dinner when you are alone at home; adding protein powder to ice cream and calling it a meal; what are or were your food rituals?

Now write what you think you want at those times. Connection? Not to be bored? To wipe out old memories? To take away fear of the future? See if you can identify what the rituals of food frenzy are asking for, what they want, what they need.

Get Real with Food

Breakfast of whole foods. You will eventually find a morning ritual with food that feels wholesome and that will help your body resist food frenzy all day. Let the whole food experiences lead you into breakfast adventures. Let whole food help you feel clean, strong, clear, vibrant and radiant. Choose pure, real, whole food; eat simply, slowly, and gratefully.

Now write a new ritual or rituals that would be healing. How can you feed yourself in ways that feel nurturing? Candles and music at meals? Setting a pretty table? Trying one new recipe each week? Shopping in a new store each week to find one new fruit. What would your new rituals be?

Make a plan. Write it down.

Write what you imagine might happen if you incorporate new rituals.

Now begin to make new habits.

Chapter Thirteen

A Place of Understanding

The Infinite Goodness has such wide arms that it takes
whatever turns to it.
—Dante Aligheri

How will you hold yourself today, now that you have awakened the heart? After years of self-abandonment, I now start my days with self-acceptance. Right now, as I write, my favorite rocking chair contains me. I am held by this Shaker-type maple rocker with a beige and brown woven cotton seat. Today, after greeting the dawn, I sit in this chair for a few minutes. Daily, it welcomes me with compassion, opens its silent arms and cradles me as I sit. In my chair, there is space for all of me. I am held with a feeling of true safety and support. Memories come of being held, cradled and rocked.

I am a child.

My mother's mother, Mémère Albert, in her big overstuffed red leather rocker with antique brass studs, sits with me in the corner of her living room. Spaciousness surrounds us, as we look out the picture window to the open Atlantic Ocean. Sometimes we sing in French. Usually, we sing the same words in English, repetitively, melodically, meditatively:

Oh, the pretty baaaaa...be

Oh the pretty baaaaa...be

Her foot pushes on the floor to make the rockers go with every other syllable. "Oh, the pret-ty baaaa...be." Sometimes the chair alone and its rocking provide comfort. While I sit here, a lot happens at Mémère's house, as I am the oldest of twenty-one first cousins. Diane is the next in line, one year younger than I am. Having just made her first Holy Communion, Diane arrives one Sunday noon at Mémère's. Diane wears lace ankle socks, black patent leather shoes, and the white dress I wore last year. Delicate and pretty, it shows grass-stains now from a fall, which also resulted in tan Band-Aids up and down Diane's leg. Even as two of my aunts and my grandmother surround her, Diane's eyes redden. She cries. I can only imagine she might be feeling humiliation, shame, or embarrassment. I feel them for her, too. And I rock.

My mother's father, Pépère Albert came home from the hospital once while I visited. His usual self, he laughed, told jokes, ate Spanish peanuts. He had undergone some surgery, which I did not understand; something about his prostate. I could tell he was my Pépère from his loud voice and his joking. "Keep your plumbing in order," he teased. But he did not look like Pépère. He was even thinner than his usual wiry self. His color was white. Although Mémère took care of his every need, I imagined that skeleton was my Pépère dying. And I rocked.

Mémère Lebel, my father's mother, had a diminutive rocker with her knitting bag next to it on the floor to its right. With bent wood all around the outside, this chair's center was a little seat, which Mémère had crocheted, green background with pastel flowers in the middle. Her tiny rocker was small enough for just me alone, and big enough for my petite grandmother and me to sit and rock together. To the right of the rocker was her gray stone fireplace. In that rocker, I learned left from right. For years, I'd turn my body around into the configuration of that chair, that fireplace, that knitting bag, to know which was my right hand. Playfully, Pépère Lebel loved to teach me new words, new ideas, and when I would confuse right from left, I would beg, "Pépère, which is which?" He never told me. Smiling, he accepted my not knowing, and tenderly urged, "Let's see, how can you find out for yourself? Where's that rocker?"

> The hurt you embrace becomes joy. Call it to your arms where it can change.
> Rumi

Rocking was not so much a way of passing time in my family. It was a way to be held, a way to learn that ups and downs eventually smooth out, that life will be full of pain and joy and that we can feel supported through it all. Through sickness and emotional storms, we grew into a trust in something larger, like big arms soothing our souls.

Heartfulness is a big rocking chair.

No one tried to fix me in these rocking chairs. Only comfort and security were offered: "Oh, the pretty baby." Troubles swinging back and forth, the arms of compassionate adults and the rockers themselves honored whatever I needed in those moments and, at the very same time, would soothe me into seeing the possibility of greater happiness.

Heartfulness is a big rocking chair. Starting my grown-up day with a few minutes in the chair, I am less likely to gobble anything in sight and more likely to remember to hold myself gently as the day goes on. When I notice the heart closing, or feelings of vulnerability arise, I rock myself inwardly, open up a space to hold what's going on. Often I sit in my Shaker chair, and sing the first loving-kindness meditation I ever heard: "Oh, the Pretty Baby."

The breath rocks, and heart awareness, like the chair, honors it all. Mostly I breathe into the gut that is tight, or the throat that is closed, and especially that soft place in the middle of my chest. With heartfulness as container, breath, body, and mind rock in the spacious comfort of the place that has offered healing… opening, opening, opening, softening, softening, softening. By cradling the moment, by making room for it to be as it is, heartfulness is a giant lap, a place to sit when the storms hit. Whether or not I literally sit in the chair, that heartfulness can stop food frenzy's temper tantrums.

I start my day gently. Every day I hold myself even for just a few moments, because when I rock myself in the container of heartfulness, my life is different. I can then embrace others differently, too—with more caring for their lives and their struggles. Experiencing being held, I can then hold.

      Oh, the pretty baaaaa…be.

      Oh, the pretty baaaaa…be

Oh the pretty baaaaa…be

In rockers we learned what it is to be small and human and yet embraced by the hands of what is greater, by an intelligence that is smarter. Rocking is Mary holding Jesus. "Put your troubles in the lap of the Buddha," those who understand quieting say, or maybe "release the small to the Infinite."

Antidotes to Food Frenzy

Find Your Heart (Thirteen minutes)

Recovering from food abuse is not so much about losing weight or getting thin as it is about healing our relationship to food and our bodies. The only way not to be still crazy after all these years is to practice the opposite of crazy-making habits. Because we tend to forget, over and over again, we need to make space to remind ourselves of the power of the heart. Where will you go?

As a daily ritual, find or create a place, a space in which to learn what is under all the surface behaviors, to feel into the heart and body, to feel your wholeness, to sink into your heart for a few moments, and to remind yourself of the simplicity of real, whole plant-based foods.

Any time food obsession or compulsion starts to shake your whole being, go in your mind or go physically to a place that can rock you gently.

While you are being held, let the image of real, whole, plant-based foods come to you. Luscious fruits, green leafies, a cornucopia of other vegetables, almonds, walnuts, sunflower seeds, nutty brown rice, lentils, peas, black beans. Let the images come. Eating from nature is a skill we practice.

> Recovering from food abuse is not so much about losing weight or getting thin as it is about healing our relationship to food and our bodies.

Let your heart help you visualize the vibrancy of real food.

Any time during the day when the buzz of a banana split yells your name, or you think you might die if you don't eat that little something with its instant energy rush, stop and imagine yourself held, rocked. Be gentle. Go slow.

Right now, go to a safe place, a comfy chair, a rocker, a pillow, your own special room, or out in nature. Sit for thirteen minutes, feeling held, feeling rocked by the bigness of what is holding you, feeling whole.

Know Thyself

Renew your full nourishment list. One daily ritual we began at the start of this book, which can help you every day of your life, is your "full nourishment list." If we begin each day writing what's working in our lives, what holds us, how we feel supported, we go through the day feeling more filled and less likely to end up calling ourselves compulsive gluttons. No need. We are already full. Life is abundant. Begin again, if you have let this practice go. Right now, write.

> Love makes everything that is heavy light.
> Thomas A. Kempis

Here is part of my list today:

- I am sitting in a chair, held by the floor, held by the earth.

- I am breathing fresh, clean air.

- The electricity works.

- I have the washing machine to clean my clothes.

- My oversized soft bathrobe keeps me warm.

- I have hot water for my shower.

- The fridge kept my breakfast blueberries fresh all night.

- While I slept, I received several quotes via email from inspirational websites so I get to start my day with the motivation to take good care of myself, my relationships and my work.

- My husband is here rummaging around and I like his energy in the house.

- My beautiful white desk with pictures of my grandchildren greets me.

Now write your list.

Get Real with Food

The Bhagavad Gita (500 BC), the wisdom of the yogic tradition, spells out how to eat for health and happiness, for mental clarity, tranquility of mind, and freedom from bondage to our old habits. The *Gita* details how automatic patterns can keep us feeling either exhausted, run-down, and lethargic, or super-charged and restless. For steady energy, balance, harmony, vigor and long life, the yogis have always taught that our food should be pure, real and fresh, so as not to stiffen the body with toxins and so we can digest easily. The yogis advise us to offer what we eat to something greater than appetite or desire, and to offer it to body/mind/soul peace, to health, to lessen the suffering of I-need-a-fix so that we may all be free from the mania of chowing down.

> To keep the body in good health is a duty... Otherwise we shall not be able to keep our mind strong and clear.
>
> Buddha

Information alone does not heal. Even now that you know how the ancient yogis taught, you must take action.

Today (and if you can commit to longer, then for a week or a month) don't eat anything artificial. Eat only what might have been available when the *Bhagavad Gita* was written: figs, apples, plums, lettuce, almonds... If you have an urge to put in your mouth newly-invented food-like matter, such as salty, greasy potato chips, see what happens if you let go of what no longer works. See what happens if you forgo it today and eat with the intention to create peace in your body and mind. That natural intelligence of the body and the garden will hold you physically, emotionally, mentally and spiritually. The garden is a huge rocking chair.

Chapter Fourteen
Choosing Food Heartfully

No more advice. Let yourself be silently drawn
by the stronger pull
of what you really love.

—Rumi

So many diets. So many theories. The mind wants to choose foods perfectly (whatever "perfect" is), as if eating right all the time (whatever "right" is) would be a magic pill. Believing there was safety in some special food plan that someone else must know, I searched for years for this illusory perfect diet. I would never age. I would never get wrinkles. I would never gain weight. I would always feel vibrant. If I bought the right supplements or the right books, or ate a certain combination of foods at certain times in certain ways, all would be well. I would live forever, I suppose. If I only knew the secret. So I bought more books, joined more classes, sought out yet another dietician, and promised over and over again, "this is it. This'll fix me for sure."

> Everybody gets so much information all day long that they lose their common sense.
> Gertrude Stein

I've adopted never-be-sick food plans and had pneumonia at the same time. I've white-knuckled a number of "perfect" diets and ended every one with pints of Rocky Road ice cream, with lots of pints of Rocky Road. It's well known that dieting causes bingeing. Hundreds of studies show that when people are put on diets, the result is food obsession, even when they had no previous history of weight or body issues. Paradoxically we come to believe that after bingeing, we must restrict. In fact, according to my personal experience and the clinical research, the opposite is true. Dieting causes bingeing. Restricting causes overeating. That's science. The body is hardwired for survival. It will not be fooled by the mind's play. Even the idea of dieting causes bingeing. Last Supper Syndrome. "Tomorrow I'll start something new. Today I eat what I will not eat ever again in my whole life starting tomorrow."

Even as I dwell in the heart, practice early morning heartfulness, and remember to return to the heart all day, still, the question remains: what do I eat? Eating lots of refined sugar is not the way to tranquility. Science also proves what those of us with sensitive systems learned long ago: junk food is not the way to strength, health and true nourishment. Acting impulsively is not freedom—it is bondage. If our compulsion chooses and we stuff ourselves with caramel corn day after day, the heart starves.

> You don't have to count every calorie if you make every calorie count.
> John Robbins

Healthy food choices make a difference. The American Heart Association, the American Cancer Association, the American Diabetes Association, and the Physician's Committee for Responsible Medicine all share similar dietary guidelines; not exact, but similar. Eat a variety of fruits and vegetables, whole grains, beans and legumes. Eliminate or limit most fats, especially saturated and trans fats. Reduce salt. Exercise. Hydrate. Increase both soluble and insoluble fiber and complex carbohydrates. Eliminate or limit simple sugars.

Antidotes to Food Frenzy

Find Your Heart (Fourteen minutes)

Heartfulness assumes that if you can ask a question, you can answer it. As soon as you hear yourself asking, "What do I eat?" focus your energy and attention to the heart. Ask your center. Listen for any answer. The heart's language will not give advice or rules. It will guide you toward what you truly love, how you will feel vibrant. You know the answer.

Choosing Food Heartfully

Go to a grocery store and spend at least fourteen minutes walking up and down the aisles.

Ask yourself, "Do I know which foods will help me feel more alive? Can I tell which foods are dead? What's really in that box? Are there any real food ingredients in that bag of candy?"

Have no intention to buy. Simply walk up and down the aisles for at least fourteen minutes and keep the attention on what you see and what happens in your heart. You'll see that you do know what to eat. You know the difference between food that is nourishing, and food that makes you feel heavy and sick. You know which not-real-foods deplete your energy. You do know that real food comes from the earth, is kissed by the sun, nourished by the soil, grown by the rain.

> Moment-to-moment heartfulness with food means staying aware, having compassion for the heart's wisdom and mustering the courage to act on it.

Does it have to be all or nothing? Ask your heart. For some of us, with some fake food stuff like flour and sugar and artificial chemicals, abstinence works. For most of us, choosing a wide variety of colorful fruits, vegetables, whole grains, nuts, seeds and beans in their whole, pure, nourishing, natural grown-from-the-ground state, makes our heart sing.

Walk around.

Feel into the body.

Take a look at candy, cake, brownies, fake vitamin drinks, fried chicken and ice cream. Note how many packages are red, yellow and orange. Food marketing experts know that these attract attention and increase impulse buys. When you see them, and notice how many of them sit on the shelves, also note what your mind does, what the body does, and then go to the heart. Moment-to-moment heartfulness with food means staying aware, having compassion for the heart's wisdom, and mustering the courage to act on it. Eventually you will sense a paradigm shift. No more advice. You will be silently drawn by the stronger pull of what you really love. You do know what to eat.

> Then God said, "I give you every seed-bearing plant on the face of the whole earth and every tree that has fruit with seed in it. They will be yours for food."
>
> Genesis 1:29 NIV

Get Real with Food

After you see all the brightly-colored boxes, bags and packages, go to the produce aisle and fill your cart with yellow, orange and red foods. Peppers, squashes, apples, oranges, bananas. What else? See what you can find. Nature provides colors so we can eat abundantly and nutritiously from the Earth. Bring the colorful produce home and see what you can cook up with them, using ideas from books listed in the bibliography, if you want. Or just get creative. Have fun. Use herbs and spices. Keep it simple. Note how filling and fulfilling these real foods are.

Know Thyself

Imagine that you are your body speaking and write a note to yourself in gratitude for the changes you are making, for all the red, yellow, orange, green, purple, blue, real, whole plant food you are eating. Let your body write about any energy changes. Let the body tell you what other changes might be helpful. Let the body write how it feels. Write from the body what is right with your choices. Love and self-compassion are better motivators than fear or judgment, so use the looking-for-what's-working habit you have cultivated in your Full Nourishment list.

Chapter Fifteen

Sacred Eating

To eat in a sacred manner we need to learn to eat from the heart. …We take in the sacred, the germ of life, like the Eucharist, in gratitude and respect… When we learn to eat from the heart we honor the stomach, not just the tongue. We are once again like children learning haltingly to feed ourselves, to nurture deep hungers in a way that heals painful longings rather than intensifies them.

—Stephen Levine, *Guided Meditations,*
Explorations and Healings

How do we learn to eat from the heart?

Those of us with food frenzy eat fast, shovel in whatever tastes good, get it over with quickly. How do we learn to take in the sacred, the germ of life, like the Eucharist?

I am seven.

I receive my First Holy Communion at St. Joseph's Church, a huge Roman Catholic cathedral. On tiptoes, I can barely reach to open the imposing heavy wooden doors adorned with polished black wrought iron handles. I remember the weeks preceding my first communion, the sacrament welcoming the class of seven-year-olds, newly-arrived at the "age of reason," into the Catholic Church. This is the greatest moment of my life to date. Two or three days a week, thirty squirming first-graders practice marching together through the main door, under a carved relief of haloed angels who usher our tiny bodies into the cavernous space. In two side-by-side lines that the Sisters of Mercy try to make straight, we hop and skip our way down the wide central aisle. My stomach flutters; these rehearsals are only a part of the build-up to the actual day. There are extra Catechism lessons, long prayers to memorize, new white patent leather shoes to break in without getting dirty. Our steps echo through the vast empty expanse while striking the shiny stone floor. As our jumpy after-school bodies become more settled, we move slowly toward the altar, light beaming through the floor-to-ceiling blue- and red-stained glass windows.

Two colorful flags hang over our heads as we enter the cathedral—one of the United States and one of the Diocese of Maine. From that farthest point in the back of the church, we see a banner hanging by the altar with the words, "Christ's life was the greatest love story of all time." For what seems to be the longest walk my short squat muscular legs have ever taken, I ponder that message all the way to the front: "The greatest love story of all time; what does that mean? … The greatest love story of all time? I don't get it. Christ didn't have a girlfriend… The greatest love story of all time. Hmmm…" Bewildered, I keep reading those words. Even though I have reached the age of reason, I do not have the ability to think metaphorically, or in symbols. I cannot understand what the priest preaches about the great Mystery, even though it is, indeed, all a mystery to me.

As we approach the altar, a statue of Jesus becomes visible. He stands in what looks like a white dress, chest exposed, revealing a pink heart. A brown wooden crucifix lay in the middle of that wide-open bleeding heart. The altar sits at the heart of the cathedral. The heart of Christ, the loving teacher, is laid bare for all to witness.

> Many persons have a wrong idea of what constitutes real happiness. It is not obtained through self-gratification but thorough fidelity to a worthy purpose.
>
> Helen Keller

The heart of the Catholic Mass is eating. Only now, so many years later, can I make the connection: eating is a sacrament. Physical food is the source of life. The how of eating has to do with gratitude and respect. Sacred eating. Food and drink are transubstantiated into life energy. Because the body digests and assimilates, we become what we eat. This is the simple healing message in the oft-repeated ritual of the Roman Catholic Mass.

After weeks of practice, the Sunday finally arrives when we take communion for the very first time. At my turn at the altar, a priest I have never met places on my tongue the little white round reminder of my connection to something greater. My classmates and I have pretended for weeks with Necco Wafer candies. The priest in all his regalia mutters total mumbo-jumbo in Latin, up-down-side-to-sides the sign of the Cross near my forehead. I feel a little scared and a lot holy. Just as I have replicated on all those Thursday afternoons, except a bit more jittery on this big day, I turn and head back to my seat, secretly scanning the church for my parents. Although we have been taught to keep our eyes down, in honor of—in honor of what I do not remember—I want to smile my front-teeth-missing grin to them. I can't find them. Nevertheless, I imagine them to be beaming proudly. In my puffy white dress, the petticoat hanging, shaky hands in newly-learned prayer position and my nervous head reverently bowing beneath a bobby-pinned lace veil, I walk back to my pew, trying not to trip. Inside my mouth, my tongue rolls around my palate, working to unstick the tasteless wafer from the roof of my mouth.

> For, after all, put it as we may to ourselves, we are all of us from birth to death guests at a table which we did not spread. The sun, the earth, love, friends, our very breath are parts of the banquet.
>
> Rebecca Harding Davis

Antidotes to Food Frenzy

Find Your Heart (Fifteen minutes)

Choose a real food. An apple. A bowl of blueberries. A mixed salad. Sit with it for at least fifteen minutes today.

As the practices lengthen, notice when you sit if the mind races off. Note also how you can bring yourself back to the heart again and again, fifty thousand times if necessary.

Open yourself to any uneasiness; it is all practice and training for impulse control.

> Always be on the lookout
> for the presence of wonder.
> E. B. White

Place the real, whole plant food in your mouth as priests offer the Host; carefully, with gratitude and respect. If this is real plant food, you are communing with nature. Can you feel the heart and feel the body welcoming food? Can eating real whole plant foods be a receiving, an embracing of Earth's holiness, a reminder of the wholeness in all of life?

For fifteen minutes, practice sacred eating as nature's bounty nourishes you.

Let your heart help you visualize the vibrancy of real food. For fifteen minutes feel your special place with life-affirming foods.

Know Thyself

After you sit and practice gentle eating, record how it feels, what you like about it, what you don't like about it. See if you can record how you feel an hour later. Is it different from how you usually eat? What calms you? What gentles you? Get out your Full Nourishment List and read it over.

Remember, stress hormones, when agitated, lead us into thinking we need a fix now and fast. When we respond with "tending and befriending" as described in Chapter Three, we relax. When our nervous system is in balance, when we feel connected to something bigger than our impulses, we can align more with Nature, both our own true nature and that of the earth. When we are in alignment, choice is easy.

How can you build support for your new choices? Most of us do not need or want food police. You might need or want pals, though. Who are the family members with whom you can share nutrient-rich recipes? Who are the friends to invite for dinner to try plant-based menus? How could you start a book group and work this book chapter-by-chapter, week-by-week, sharing your experiences? Who could be a phone buddy so you could make personal contact when needed? Can you find a plant-based dietitian in your area? Which doctors near you are learning about nutrition? Are there groups that could help you?

Get Real with Food

Some foods jolt our "needing a fix" nervous system. Coffee has caffeine. Chocolate mimics opiates. Many men report needing a burger fix. Cheese and dairy products with their caso-morphines release mild opiates during digestion. Sugar hits the same brain receptors as heroine. Meat, sugar, and cheese jazz our brains. They are not conducive to food peace, to calm mind, to body wellness, to eating in a mindful and heartful way. They are not a solution. It's easier to prevent the highs and the fog-filled lows of food frenzy than it is to intervene with it once it starts. Plant-based science teaches that a lack of nutrients in our processed food causes us to search for nutrients in addictive food-like substances.

> All nature is at the disposal of mankind. We are to work with it. Without it we cannot survive.
> Hildegard of Bingen

Today choose lots of fruits and vegetables, whole grains, legumes and a few nuts and seeds with lots of fiber, antioxidants, phytonurients. Notice if these new behaviors and choices diminish gotta-have-it food frenzy and overeating junk. We increase what works and decrease what hurts us and then we pay attention to how we feel. Plant-based dieticians tell us that if we eat more than 90 percent of our diets from whole, real, natural plant foods, our health on all levels will soar.

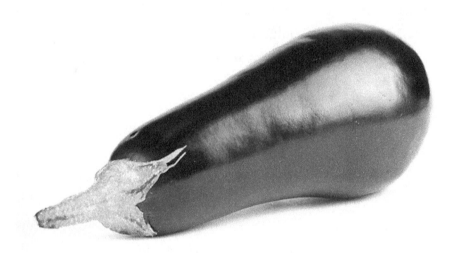

Chapter Sixteen

Beauty...

The
gift of
lightness arrives not in
pounds, but in
heart.
Body obsession, not
beauty, is skin deep.
—Susan Lebel Young

I was not always this self-nurturing. I did not always know the difference be-tween taking food and receiving nourishment. Heartfulness necessitates find-ing interests beyond self-destruction. So my early morning practices now also include feeling into my body, moving into my being, in ways that invite some-thing more meaningful, more pleasurable, and ultimately more nutritious than going for the burn. My earlier obsession for high-level fitness, certainly normal in this fat-phobic culture, has transformed into wanting high-level wellness, which includes physical, emotional, spiritual and mental fitness. In this cul-ture, eating enough processed food to reach food coma, needing antacids, wak-ing up with food hangovers and then pounding it out at the gym to make up for it are culturally accepted behaviors.

I am forty-eight.

One day, in the fall of her senior year of high school, Alisa returns home from field hockey practice exhausted. As she collapses on the sofa, I ask what sort of drills the team did today. Jokingly, Alisa chides me that they were drills for eighteen-year-olds only, and lists off crosses and tips, running relays and sprints. She mentions that the girls did forty push-ups during the course of the practice. As if a gauntlet has been thrown, I spring into action. Without hesitation, I turn off the burner on which I have been sautéing onions, drop to the kitchen floor and exclaim that I am not as old as she thinks. Forget dinner preparation: I do forty push-ups. "You know, Alisa," I tease, "I have the wisdom of a fifty-year-old in an eighteen-year-old body."

By the next afternoon, my shoulder is completely covered in tape and wrapped in a splint from physical therapy. Laughing, I point out to Alisa that this decision to dive into so many pushups clearly reflects the wisdom of an eighteen year-old in a almost fifty-year-old body. The bursitis lasts months. Three years later, I still have residual weakness and sensitivity in the anterior deltoid and coracobrachialis of the right arm, but I am fit, damn it.

Bodies never lie.
Agnes De Mille

A lifetime drive for thinness and muscularity takes its toll. Dying to be skinny eclipses healthy self-care. It is one thing to want to be healthy, agile, have strong bones, or more energy. These are the healthy intentions, which I would eventually learn from yoga. For years they played only a minimal role in my conditioning craze. I wanted body sculpture. From a seductive media ad, I sent away for a program called, "Eliminate Ab Flab." I learned words like "internal and external obliques." I did not care that these muscle fibers, running in various directions around my belly, were responsible for side bending. I could not see the great intelligence in the body: I simply did not want love handles. Period. It did interest me that bilateral contraction of these obliques causes compression of the abdomen. Compression of the abdomen must be good, I figured. Nor was I interested in the function of the obliques in assisting in flexion of the trunk. I had my values. I also became obsessed with the transversus abdominis, the circular fibers running around the waist, which, when contracted, reduce the diameter of the abdomen. I pulled in my belly so hard for so long that my back ached all the time. No matter: I was on my way to ripped abs. According to this "Eliminate Ab Flab" tape, the long *rectus abdominus* was a flexor for the trunk, but it also assists in compressing the abdomen. Crunches. Sit-ups. This vertical sheath was on its way to being tight (which was the goal—right?—regardless of my tension and stiffness in the lower back). Little did I know then that the best way to a healthy back is to allow the belly to move while breathing. Letting the abdominal organs soften in order to breathe in ways that release tension never occurred to me. Even the purpose of powerful abs to support the spine in suppleness and resilience was lost in the quest for "lookin' good."

I rendered the same abuse with the flabby thighs I hated; sculpt and tone, even thought "Butt Blasters" was a good idea. Perhaps the saddest injury in this pursuit of sleek and taught was the violation of the natural rhythm of breathing. Sucking in through the stomach tightens the diaphragm, thereby restricting breath, allowing less oxygen to circulate. This refusal to "fill up" cuts off life energy. We bind our body energy in a corset. The muscles of respiration—the internal and external intercostals, the levatores costarum, the transverses thoracis, and the diaphragm—are intended to move freely with normal inhalation and exhalation. When there is conflict between externally imposed aesthetics and breathing, routine activities like speaking, coughing and eating are all affected. This tummy tucking meant I could not eat that one raisin when I first read the work of Jon Kabat-Zinn and tried his mindful eating suggestions. For years I had sat at a table taking in food but constricting breath all the while, destroying any possibility of true nourishment—physical oxygen, or the spiritual life force.

I am a genetically muscular person. Muscularly built, tight, compressed. Muscularly firm, stable. Muscularly fit. My habit is to move with a sense of my musculoskeletal structure, lifting weights, walking strong. But there is more to a whole person than muscular energy, and ultimately the healing from food hell celebrates the body from the

> Volumes are now written and spoken about the effect of the mind upon the body. Much of it is true. But I wish a little more was thought of the effect of the body on the mind.
>
> Florence Nightingale

inside and from the core, which is deeper than the musculature on the surface.

I am fifty-five.

In a yoga class, I sit behind other yoginis and cannot see Rebecca, the teacher, as she demonstrates a pose. I want to get it right. As I wriggle across the floor to assure myself a better view, Rebecca laughs at me. "What are you doing, Sue?"

"I can't see you."

She chuckles, "Good! Yoga guides us to move from the inside out."

I did not understand then. But it planted a seed, seeds now watered in daily gentle stretching practice. Relaxing effort, focusing on spiritual fitness, letting go of the intense focus on the physical, celebrating wholeness from the inside out.

> Healing from food hell celebrates the body from the inside and from the core, which is deeper than the musculature on the surface.

I am in college.

When I teach skiing, the leaders of the ski school check our "finished forms." We need to perform our turns with impeccable precision. Every few weeks a videographer focuses on each instructor separately as we make our way down an open slope, filming every turn. Later, we review the film and give each other feedback. The very first time the tape runs, I do not see my lovely form, exact unweighting and timely pole-plant. The instant I see my yellow pants and navy parka on the screen, I let out an impulsive scream, "Oh, my God, I really am short and fat."

Sometimes I still catch myself judging my outsides like that. But, since Rebecca's reminder and the practices of heartfulness, I am experiencing a new kind of seeing, a new kind of "lookin' good."

I am fifty-six.

I review a videotape of a yoga class that I teach. There is no familiar clenching of the jaw as the tape begins to roll, no increased heart rate, or fist in the gut. Simply watching, I look for the details of my teaching. Chuckling to myself, I note that years ago I would have wondered if purple was the right color to wear for such an event. This time I do not look at my hair or my belly but observe how I teach postures, how my voice sounds. Affirming that I like the tone and quality of my voice, I can admit that it sounds soft, accepting, nurturing and clear. I observe how often I smile and note that the teacher is (I am) smiling. This version of myself seems to improvise, relax and have fun. I see my strengths in giving lots of permission for beginning students to explore, make it their own. I include the students in the process. The biggest thrill for me is to see the transformation in my style—from the brute force of "going for the burn" to gently coaxing the vital force, inviting it to come through me, encouraging it to come forth in the students. I feel kindness towards myself when I see those places of discomfort in the video, my reluctance to push people, my hesitancy in teaching certain postures. I make a simple mental note to learn more about a few nuances: the balance of verbal instruction and the time given to move; the introduction of counter-poses; and to watch alignment in people more carefully. I watch and feel thankful for this shift in my perception of what it means to be healthy and well.

I am not judging fitness programs; I work with a trainer. Joe challenges me to stay strong, to maintain bone density, to have good range of motion. I walk most days and practice yoga. Working out is good. So is "working in." There is nothing wrong with wanting to be fit, lean and healthy. But my quest for what I thought ripped abs would give me now has a different intention. The old motivation was "how buff can I be?" My question is now, "can I enter a movement experience with an attitude of gratitude, out of self-love rather than self-flagellation?" Instead of yet another physical self-improvement campaign, can I see exercise as I see food—more holistically?

I am a being far greater than I have yet conceived. I am unfolding gradually but surely...moving forward and upward constantly.

Yogi Ramacharaka

Antidotes to Food Frenzy

Find Your Heart (Sixteen minutes)

It seems reasonable when we read the flyers: "Six-Pack Abs by Christmas." The trainer-to-be advertises that she wants her former hard body back. We can join her for sit-ups and variations for a half-hour three times a week. In three months we are promised much-coveted midriffs-of-steel.

We sign on. The first day we walk into the gym, we see that some men and women crunching away might indeed have flat stomachs by the holidays. For us, we wonder how we ever deemed all this grunting a good idea.

> If anything is sacred, the human body is sacred.
> Walt Whitman

We do the sets of clean crunches, oblique circles and cross-over reaches. We suck our bellies in and up and breathe as the trainer instructs; shallow, rapid, short. "Focus on the exhale, navel to spine, abdomen in and up."

She barks orders: "Two more reps; go for it."

We go for it.

But we can't tighten the rib cage and torso and still breathe fully. If we pull hard in and up, how do we let down? How do we take it easy?

Today let's practice what AIDS worker, meditation instructor, and poet Stephen Levine calls Soft Belly, a way to calm the nervous system, a way to learn to stay in the bodies we have rather than wish they were different, a way to practice long, slow, deep, gentle breathing, all ways to help with grab-and-go food fix. You can't have soft belly and feel food frenzy at the same time.

Here's how to practice Soft Belly: Let the muscles around the waist relax. Let the in-breath enter the body and go down into a soft belly. Deep, slow, long breaths. Each in-breath raises the abdomen and expands the musculature. We round, make space. With each exhale, the abdomen falls, the strain of up-tight dispels.

Here's what I've learned with Soft Belly practice: to go through life with ease, facing joy and pain, yours and others, you may have to practice Soft Belly ten thousand times a day. Inhale down into the belly. Exhale past the heart. The softer the belly, the more we can stay present and awake. The culture crunches us into hard-belly. Yet to be fully alive, we can both train our abs physically and then soften the belly and deepen the breath to ease our minds and open our hearts.

When you choose to exercise: start by getting down on the floor and practice Soft Belly for a few minutes and move in ways that feel right to the body. Let go of any idea of needing to know a perfect stretch or do so many sets and reps. Let the body lead. Listen to what it wants. Maybe gentle rocking. Maybe full body stretches, maybe head rolls. Simply listen. Trust gut feelings. Your true center will start to talk to you when you drop your attention out of your head and into your core and feel into your body.

For sixteen minutes today, with as much gratitude as you can muster for this body which has seen you through all these years, sit with Soft Belly practice.

Know Thyself

Appropriate exercise and movement that match our body, temperament and health are stepping stones on the path of heartfulness. When we honor, rather than beat up or give up on our bodies, we can see more clearly the mind-habits of self-doubts, fears and judgments. Some of us are emotionally attached to overdoing exercise. Others of us are emotionally attached to sitting on the sofa all day. The heart does not know extremes. We can learn to trust the unfolding beauty and wisdom in each cell if we pay attention and clear a channel to the heart.

> Your true center will start to talk to you when you drop your attention out of your head and into your core and feel into your body.

How will you begin to comprehend that each life is precious, including your own?

How will you find the inspiration to be fully present to its real needs in each moment?

What will you choose for your heartful movement? Gentle yoga? Tai chi? Short or long walks? Running? Biking? Lifting weights? Something competitive like tennis? Ask your body and heart… you may be surprised at what you hear.

Go to your heart.

Ask.

Listen for the heart's answer.

Pay attention.

Can you follow what the heart has to say?

Go to your journal. Write for sixteen minutes. Consider offering deep gratitude for your body.

Get Real with Food

Our bodies, too, are ancient. By design, some foods increase the stress on the body. Some foods keep us healthy and strong both physically and mentally. Some foods help us maintain the body at the weight we are supposed to be. Some foods help us reduce body fat, boost energy, enhance mood, cut the need for a sugar-fix. That's good news, because the human body has evolved through the millennia to function best on the fuel provided by nature. Whole real plant foods fuel our body for movement, for energy, for getting through the day, for exercise.

Notice the difference in your motivation to work out (or "work-in") when you have coffee, donuts, eggs and sausage for breakfast or when you start the day with a bowl of oats topped with apple, cinnamon and walnuts.

Notice how you feel after a lunch of burger, fries and a milk shake or when you have a huge salad and a bean soup. Note the difference in your energy when you have a steak and macaroni and cheese for dinner or a huge veggie stir-fry with brown rice.

Try out low-fat, whole food, plant-based eating and note what happens to your exercise regimen and regularity due to the presence or lack of food hangover in the morning.

The student asks:
"Grant me some great wisdom. What is the most important thing?"
The teacher replies,
"Attention."
"Is there more?"
"Attention. Attention."
Zen story

Chapter Seventeen

Softening the Heart

We read that we ought to forgive our enemies
But we do not read that we ought to forgive our friend.
                                        —Cosimo de Medici

I am thirty-nine.

The ring of the phone awakens me at 6:30 a.m. It's Dad. He's been up all night; waited until now to call. "Susan, Meghan is dead. She died in her sleep last night. Paul will be here if you want to come over."

Paul is my baby brother; Meghan, his infant daughter.

Driving to my parents' home, my mind floods with Paul's life story. It has been full of struggle.

Paul and Peter were twins, born eight weeks premature. They suffered severe medical complications through the birth process, including oxygen deprivation. Both less than three pounds at birth, their lungs were not fully developed. As a sixteen-year-old, I visited my forty-two-year-old Mom two days after the birth at Mercy Hospital. I held her weak arm, helping her hobble from her maternity room so we could peek through the nursery window at her newborn twin sons, her seventh and eighth children. Six-feet tall, Dr. Good gently picked up the tiny preemies, placed one in each of his encompassing palms, and brought them close for Mom to see.

One day when we arrived, Peter was blue. My mother gasped and stifled tears. She used one hand to grip my arm, the other to cover her face, "Oh, my God," she shrieked, "He's not dead is he?"

Not that time. The pediatric nurse rushed to suction his lungs and Peter survived that day. But he didn't make it. Peter died after only a couple of days. Now my mother had seven children to care for. Six waiting at a home, and a very needy newborn.

As far as I know, with the code of my mother's era and generation, she could never allow herself to grieve the loss of that baby or the others she had lost in the womb and in stillbirths. Or the death of her older sister who died of breast cancer at a young age. My mother got busy, smoked a lot of cigarettes and pretended it didn't hurt.

Paul came home from the hospital, alone without his "womb mate." Fairly soon we noticed the developmental lags that characterize what was then labeled minimal brain damage. Early speech problems, multiple learning disabilities, hyperactivity. He received sympathy, pity, drugs, and lots of "special help." Paul nevertheless struggled with learning to read and write, with focus in school, with making and keeping friends, with completing dinner without spilling his milk. Life was hard for him as a kid.

Even his marriage was tough—sudden, as the result of an unplanned pregnancy—then full of conflict in those first stressful months. But when Meghan arrived, she seemed to make everything better. Meghan had been the light of Paul's life. He beamed when he held her as she gurgled and cuddled into his thick, broad neck. For three months Paul had thrived on the new identity of "Daddy," as he joined his six older siblings as "parent."

He already had so much to grieve in his young life, and now at twenty-three, his three-month-old daughter has just died of Sudden Infant Death Syndrome. Paul had put Meghan in her crib last evening healthy—big fat rosy-red cheeks, big round wide-open blue eyes, smiling, laughing and cooing. Early this morning he had been the one to find her in that crib motionless, blue-black, not breathing. He administered CPR, called an ambulance, and continued with CPR until help arrived. But she was already gone.

By 9:00 a.m., I pull into Mom and Dad's driveway. Even as I open the door to the back hallway, I catch a whiff of the burning smoke I know to be my mother's cigarette. I also note the salty, smoky smell, clearly identifiable as deli ham. In the kitchen, my father paces the floor holding a pen and piece of paper in this hands. Mom stands at the counter slicing generic-brand white bulky rolls. Lots of turmoil. No eye contact. The room fills with heavy silence, yet the confusion and disbelief are palpable. Dad sits at the kitchen table, ready to write, and uttered, "Sue, sit here and help me think of some nice families we might invite to join the country club. Membership just opened up."

Ignoring him, Mom orders, "Help me with the food. Put the cold cuts on the platter."

"Oh, my God," I scream to myself. My gut sickens, my heart closes and my internal talk intensifies. "They are so busy, so numbed. What is going on? Why is no one with Paul? He has suffered so many losses in his life and no one can sit with him?"

My emotions run high and wild. As if just punched in the stomach, I am furious with my parents. How can they be so insensitive and unreasonable? In shock about Meghan, I tremble, because in a few moments I will see my baby brother for the first time since it happened. What will I say? What will I do?

Years before, I would have jumped in, helped with the food, the whole time stuffing fistfuls of white dinner rolls and Reese's cups into my chomping jaw. The buffet has already been organized, so easy to attack: bits of iceberg, packaged slaw, pineapple chunks packed in their own juice, King Cole vinegar-and-salt potato chips, and store brand peanut butter chip cookies, the kind that bend when you try to break off a piece. Surely being busy with the external act of chewing would quiet the internal horror. I used to eat to numb myself. It's all I knew.

This time I use my breath to soften the belly, and I sink into my heart, still not knowing what to say to Paul. I don't want to make stupid chatter. I want simply to be with him. Just to be, just to sit, just to offer presence. Yet I put off seeing Paul, incredulous about Meghan, and outraged at my parents. No matter that I am immobilized; my mind nevertheless screams internally, "What the hell is going on here?"

I manage to blurt, "Where's Paul?"

My parents pace and prepare the house for guests. Mom makes coffee; Dad moves furniture to accommodate the anticipated crowd. As he shakes his head, I hear him mumble, barely audibly, "You can understand death when it's an adult, but how do you make sense of it when it's an infant?"

When they finally look up at me, I see that their eyes are red and puffy. A wave of compassion washes over me; they are human beings, doing the best they can in this horrible situation. They are giving all they have. How quickly I judged. How little I knew what has happened in this house in the past few hours. My first reaction was to assume whatever they were doing was not enough. My barriers to compassion crumble now and empathy floods the moment. Looking at their paralysis, I see that we are the same in our confusion and pain. None of us knows what to do. In this instant, all my resentments melt. For the first time, I see tears in their eyes and feel their humanity.

It is only with the heart that one can see rightly: what is essential is invisible to the eye.
Antoine de Saint-Exupéry

My own heart opens. I relax and go to Paul. Tears start in the kitchen and flow by the time I find Paul in the master bedroom. As I hold him, I cry, not knowing what to say. He repeats again and again, "This sucks." While we sit on the bed, we cry together. We hold hands. We hug. We rock in each other's embrace. We remain in silence, except for the sobs.

In the Buddhist and yogic practices of friendliness toward others and ourselves, often called lovingkindness, we are asked to open our hearts to what is most challenging. This day I was called to "keep the heart open in hell." The pain of my closed and judging heart might have kept me from fully being with Paul. My old habit of "stuff down food to stuff down feelings" might have led me to numbing the horror of the day. Eventually, with time, patience and practice, we come to open the heart and we stop using food to fix what cannot be fixed.

Antidotes to Food Frenzy

Find Your Heart (Seventeen minutes)

What's in your heart?

Sit.

Stop.

Take a breath.

Feel into the heart. Even if you feel nothing, still, having the intention to open the heart begins to teach us how to feel. Heartfulness, coming into the heart, seeing from the heart, will help us be with the toughest stuff in life knowing we can't fix it, knowing nothing needs to be fixed. Heartfulness is like an anchor in the middle of a storm. It grounds us. It steadies us. We can learn to feel and accept what is. We can sit with our emotions. We can be. Life's roughest times are already full enough.

See if you can sit here for seventeen minutes, in your heart, feeling into your core. Note the times you want to get up and do something else, anything else. This is normal. Then sit a little more. The practices of heartfulness, if they are to help us reduce our impulsive gimme-that-now, need to challenge us to stretch beyond our comfort zone just a little each time. Sit. Stay. Feel. Stay longer than you think you could. You can.

> We are healed of our suffering only by experiencing it to the full.
> Marcel Proust

Know Thyself

What are the times you are most likely to get triggered to want to eat what we often call "comfort foods?" (Have you noticed they don't comfort in the long run?) Under what kinds of stress do you want to fix life with food? Where do you get stuck and want to slip into automatic pilot eating? You have been practicing sitting with what is for seventeen minutes. Notice any improvement in impulse control as a result. **Write about any changes in you.**

Get Real with Food

Under stress, the body burns carbohydrates, fats and B vitamins. Under stress, the hunger signals shut down, as does digestion, so blood can shunt to the extremities to get us ready to run or fight. The stress hormones are high in the body. Adrenaline rushes. Cortisol spikes. When the stress resolves, the stress hormones come back into balance but cortisol stays high to increase our appetites so we can refuel. This is normal. This is natural. It is not that there is something wrong with us. There is nothing to fix. We are not bad. The body has its own brilliant intelligence. With its signals it tries to teach us to stay well-fueled with complex carbohydrates: fruits, vegetables, grains, beans. We need these for our brains and clear thinking, to nourish our muscles and bodies.

Try adding more fruits, vegetables, whole grains and beans. When we stay nourished with real, whole plant foods, the body stays in balance better and longer.

> You must do the thing you think you cannot do.
> Eleanor Roosevelt

Can you add a whole grain to every meal? Try it and see if it helps with stress management and craving control.

Chapter Eighteen

Feeling Feelings

Life is the only real counselor.
—Edith Wharton

I am fifty.

It is Sunday. I receive a call from my friend Reid. He asks, "Are you sitting down?"

"No," I say, and chuckle to myself because of his choice of the old cliché.

"Well, you'd better sit," his voice is somber.

"Why?" I want to know.

I don't sit, as I am still walking around my kitchen "multi-tasking"—opening the fridge, turning on a burner, starting water to boil, removing the morning paper from the table, choosing tea, and holding the phone. Reid must assume I am sitting, as he tells me, "Alex is dead…Alex died today."

I sit, no, drop, onto the hard wooden chair.

I met Alex in the early 1990s, full of life, handsome with shocking white hair and thick black eyebrows, an endearing Scottish brogue, laughing, talking, eyes sparkling, always knowing when to tease and when to drop the fun and go compassionately deep, being supportive in either case. From Alex, I learned clinical pastoral skills, people skills, how to be with human beings without trying to fix them, how to walk together with people through the worst pain or suffering of their lives, how to speak truth about myself, how to open to others and how to punctuate any moment with a good joke.

I dismiss Reid's news. Alex was only sixty-something. Reid's story is bizarre. How could Alex drop dead instantly of a heart attack in the middle of an energetic tennis game? As far as I know, Alex doesn't even play tennis. With firm refusal to believe, I am aware of no feelings—nothing other than a fierce curiosity to discover how such a wild tale could be circulating.

At first I sit, numbed about what to do next. Call Alex expecting to hear him laugh about this outrageous yarn? No, I have enough respect for Reid's integrity not to test him. After I thank Reid and hang up, the phone begins to ring. Friends start to call. It is true. Without my ever having said good-bye to Alex, without a recent thank you for all he has done for me, my dear friend and teacher is dead.

So is everything I have been learning—twenty years of meditation and stillness practice, sixteen years of psychotherapy for "the food thing," five years of graduate school to become a licensed clinical mental health counselor, the knowledge from hundreds of books on eating disorders and disordered eating, fifteen years of training to re-parent myself, even as I parent my children.

I want to cram my face with food. I want what is true not to be true. I want things to be different than they are. I want Alex and all he embodied—sweetness, intelligence, humor and skill. I am scared, sad, angry, lonely and confused, and I madly begin seeking food. I cannot sit any longer. I jump into the car.

I drive a well-honed route, fully intending to act out a very old pattern— wolfing down purchases from one store as I tear toward the next. I drive, music cranked up, racing, trying to shut out shock. I get Sunspire chocolate-covered peanuts from the Whole Grocer (Alex would have joined me. He loved eating what his diabetes would forbid). I buy chocolate and peanut butter Think Bars with gingko from the Natural Grocer (Alex's biggest fear was that he would lose his quick mind and sharp wit as he aged. He would have approved of ginko). I grab a pint of Ben & Jerry's Phish Food from Shop 'n Save (Alex might have offered me some compassionate statement at this point about his struggles with food, too). I buy a can of Planter's Dry Roasted Peanuts and a thin green box of after diner mints. My clammy hands surge toward Wheat Thins, but recoil.

I do not eat. Something stops me. An intelligent, blessed voice of the heart says, "Susan, bingeing is not going to fix this. You are not going to help the hurt with what is in these cardboard boxes and plastic wrappers. You cannot gulp food fast enough to slow the tears. You cannot eat enough to stop the grief. This is big, much bigger than sugar." Finally, I sit, sweating.

Heartfulness puts the brakes on and offers me a different choice, the choice to live fully, to feel. The deluge of tears lets loose, the rage surfaces, and the body lets go into sobbing. I cry a long time, and then Alex's face appears.

Alex once challenged me with a puzzle. Writing some letters on the blackboard, he asked with his lilting Scottish devilishness, "What does this say?"

...N...O....W.....H.....E.....R.....E.....

"No where," I had answered, in the same tone with which I might have said, "Duuuuh."

> No food can remove pain. No frantic activity will erase grief.

With a twinkling light in his eye and a playful lift of his dark brow, as if to say "gotcha," he chuckled. "That's what most people say. It can also be read 'now here.' It might be interesting for you to have a look into how you see things."

He erased the letters.

"Just a thought," he teased.

Alex's teachings come to me when I have no strength of my own. He says, "Be here, now. Stop and have a look." I do. It hurts. Feelings come. Thanks to Alex's voice, I open. Alex's sparkle helps me sit with restlessness, anger, sadness and loneliness.

No food can remove this pain. No frenetic activity will erase Alex's death. Sitting in the now-here, no longer running on old automatic pilot, I do not want to self-destruct in an attempt to numb out this death. As I feel the comfort of Alex's magical words, I receive one more gift from Alex, a favorite expression of his.

"With all the pain in the world, the work of opening the heart to it may seem like a drop in the bucket. But at least it's a drop in the right bucket."

If we practice heartfulness over and over and over, when we first wake up in the morning, when we sit to eat, when we commune with others in conversations, whenever we think of it, we come to see that heartfulness is a skill. We build it through practice. Only if we practice again and again will heartfulness come to us in those I-can't-stand-this moments, stressful times when we most need our hearts. When heartfulness becomes a habit and replaces old automatic patterns, it comes when we need help, inspires us, and keeps us awake. Heartfulness can take our hands out of the cookie jar, keep our arms out of the fridge, and support us in managing every "now here" no matter how unmanageable life may seem.

Antidotes to Food Frenzy

Find Your Heart (Eighteen minutes)

Stop. Move your attention to the middle of your chest.

Notice what you feel there. Even if you feel nothing, see if you can rest your awareness in your very core. Feel into your body. Like grains of sand falling in an hourglass, let your weight go into gravity. Feel into your heart. Heartfulness can be called forth even in the midst of illness and death. We can be "now here" with warmth and comfort toward ourselves and others if we stay in close to the heart.

Sit here now for eighteen minutes simply resting in the heart. You may feel bored or "never in a million years can I do this." That's the giddy-up mind talking. The heart wants more, wants us to be able to sit with fears, doubts and anger without a trip to Burger Palace.

Then, after you finish these eighteen minutes, see about maintaining a

> Heartfulness can take our hands out of the cookie jar, keep our arms out of the fridge, and support us in managing every "now here" no matter how unmanageable life may seem.

connection to this life-giving center as often as you can all day. Heartfulness will keep you in touch with your inner resources and the movement of vital energy flowing in your body.

Stay. Feel. Notice.

Bring any ease pumped by the heart with you as you move on.

> It makes me laugh to read over this diary. It's so full of contradictions and one would think I was such an unhappy woman. Yet is there a happier woman than I?
>
> Sophie Tolstoy

Know Thyself

Now that you have practiced sitting and eating great food and knowing your story, **write in your Full Nourishment list what is truly satisfying.** What are those things in your life that will endure longer than a Diet Coke? What is sustainable over time to help you be fully well, vibrant, radiant and whole? Can you feel into a deep body connection to what is deeply steadying and satisfying?

Get Real with Food

Take some real food to a table. An apple. A salad. A snack or a meal. Begin to pay attention to what is here, now in front of you. As you sit, visualize the farmers who grew the food to become part of your nourishment. Visualize the gardening, the harvesting, the transporting of this food that is about to go from outside your body to inside to nurture you and become you. As you eat, can you feel with all your senses? How do the colors look? Take in the smells. Feel the textures. Without awareness when we eat, whether alone or with others, we often forget we have eaten. If we grab a quick bite and stuff it down while in the car, we may have no memory of eating. Savor. Dine. Honor the food and your body as it receives, ingests, digests, assimilates. Taste. Enjoy. Appreciate and give yourself the pleasure of feeling fed, of feeling nourished. This is an antidote to food frenzy. Awareness heals.

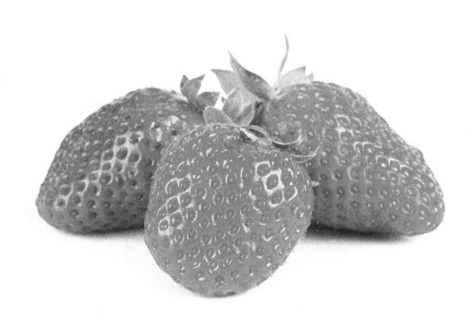

Part Four

Silence

There is a way between voice and presence
where information flows.
In disciplined silence it opens.
With wandering talk it closes.

—Rumi

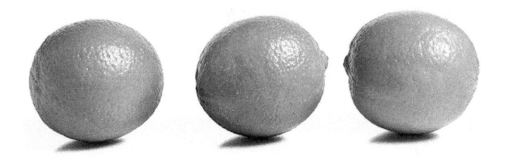

Chapter Nineteen
The Attitude of Silence

In the attitude of silence the soul finds the path in a clearer light, and what is elusive and deceptive resolves itself into crystal clearness. Our life is a long and arduous quest after Truth.

—Mahatma Gandhi

There is no separation between where this book began and where it now begins to end. The quest for awakening to something bigger than food frenzy led me to practices of the heart. Breathing empty. Breathing full. Celebrating the dawn. Rocking. Yoga. Spiritual fitness. Sacred eating. Self-acceptance. Befriending myself. Ultimately, they all taught me the beauty of silence, which I learned as a child from my big, blue Casco Bay. These practices collectively teach a way of living in the world. In that sense, they are not techniques. Though I do not do them perfectly (whatever that is) or have consistent results (whatever they would be), this awakening to the heart is more a way of being than a perfunctory performance of exercises.

Just as there was struggling in the beginning because I wanted the practices to work (whatever that means), now I teach others to go to their silent oceanic place inside, however that makes sense for them. In classes for meditation or yoga, or in private sessions, I leave places of silence, gaps in which the wisdom appears.

I am fifty-six.

After my yoga class, in which I lead a few quiet deep-cleansing breaths to help him hold the grief of his grandfather's passing, Joe says, "It was the stillness in the room that last night of his life that was so powerful. We were all there; twenty of his closest relatives came to say 'goodbye.' I did not know what to say, so I was quiet and held his hand. That silence meant everything. Now I understand it. Thank you for the long silence in class tonight."

I want to respond. Instead I hold the quiet, to honor his hushed tones.

Rita finds me after class, silently wiping away tears. She says, "I was caught off guard by my emotions when you talked about the power of silence. I was so touched and moved by people coming together through pain and how, in the silence of the class, we all cared for each other. That silence was healing for me."

Again, I want to talk. Again, I stay quiet.

Another student, Gail, reports, "The more I build silence into my day, the stronger, clearer and more focused my intuition is. I am seeing that I do not always need all the words I usually use to be in touch with people. Communication becomes more efficient."

As teacher, as therapist, as student of silence, my old habitual way is to want to speak. My challenge is to be still, to learn from my students, from clients and from the silence itself.

Antidotes to Food Frenzy

Find Your Heart (Nineteen minutes)

By now, if you've been practicing, you have seen how the mind will pull us out of the heart; how we need constant practice to traction us back to center. Today sit for nineteen minutes. You may notice moments of bliss, joy, insight, and moments of pain, fear, restlessness, fatigue. The heart can hold them all. You can do it, if you've been practicing. If we repeatedly go to the heart, most of us begin to notice a pleasantness where we can stay, a pleasantness that is quiet and silent and can protect us from the noise in our heads and the frenzy of looking for love in all the wrong places. Love, peace and well-being dwell in the heart. Again and again, stop, rest in your center.

Sit now for nineteen minutes and imagine the radiance of your heart first coursing through your tissues, organs, bones and muscles and then silently going out and reaching others.

> Nothing can bring you peace but yourself.
> R. W. Emerson

Know Thyself

Write how things have changed for you. With all this practice, how much more able are you to understand your feelings and their meanings for you? As you live more from the heart, how much more nurturing have you been in relationships? How has your compassion for yourself and others changed? Now that you have slowed down, learned to savor your food and changed your food consumption habits, how do you feel physically, emotionally, mentally, spiritually?

Get Real with Food

Sit with your food, quietly. If you sit quietly with various foods, you will see that some, those intended by nature for the human body, are plants, grown from Earth. If you sit with meat or fish, feel into your heart and feel into the animals' hearts. Sit with the silence of the images you see. You may feel pain for the brutal way animals are caged and medicated, for their inhumane killing, for the deaths caused them for our pleasures. When we bring our awareness to the heart and look at a bag of industrially-concocted Cheetos, we see there is no heart, only chemicals. Heartfulness, deep and quiet, makes food choices easier. When we ask the questions of the heart and listen silently for the answers, we know what feels most nourishing for us, for the animals, for the planet.

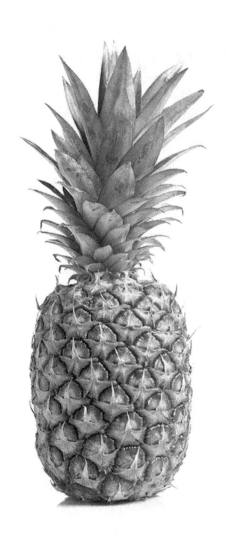

Chapter Twenty

Conscious Moments

Vitality shows in not only the ability to persist
but the ability to start over.

—F. Scott Fitzgerald

How is it, I have wondered, that I have not only lost fifty pounds and maintained that loss for almost forty years, but also have felt an ever-increasing freedom from food frenzy? How is it that I continue to insist on moving to the heart after countless obliterated days? I think I am closer to the answer now.

I used to think success was daily exercise and a low-fat, high fiber diet. But with any binge, I can instantaneously leave these both behind. The diet clubs promote going to meetings and staying to hear the message, but meetings and messages often leave me confused, or, worse yet, angry. Dieticians and coaches tout research that shows that a person needs one-to-one consultation and support. But I rebel. External authorities and I clash.

I have broken all the rules. I am a one-person disproof of all the research. For me, stepping out of a junk-food-crazy cycle happens only in present moments. Thankfully, I have been led to one conscious moment, and then one conscious moment, and then another. Again and again. Right now. This moment. This choice. Now. Here. No waiting until tomorrow morning to start over. Not beginning a new diet on Monday. We awaken to consiousness as soon as we can. Now.

I am thirty-nine.

Alisa and I decide to run a few errands at the local mall. At 9:30 a.m., we walk through the main entrance and immediately smell the bittersweet aroma of freshly-baked chocolate chip cookies. We stand directly across from Mrs. Field's inviting kiosk filled with delicious, rich, chunky, chewy, moist cookies.

My whole being responds to the sights of the little round goodies, the smell of the buttery sweetness, the memories they evoke of Mémère Lebel's baking. Lost in this euphoria I look up as Alisa's voice pulls me out of my reverie.

"I want one of those." She turns to the clerks and asks, "Could I have just one of those chocolate chunk cookies?"

The clerk replies, "We only sell them in bags of six, twelve, or twenty-four."

Furrowing her brow, Alisa turns to me as if asking what to do.

I adore chocolate chip cookies. I binge on them, and then two minutes later promise never to eat them ever again. Ever. I give myself permission to eat boxes of them, and then swear off. I get permissive with myself and then rigid. Chocolate chip cookies do this to me; or rather I go unconscious with them often.

Swept by impulsivity, I answer, "Get twenty-four. We'll take some home to Dad and Zac."

At 9:30 am, after a nutritious breakfast, we start. She eats one. I eat lots. I don't count. By the time I realize what is happening, most of the bag is gone. When I wake up from this hand-to-mouthing, I want to hide, find a way to get rid of what I have ingested, and never eat cookies again in my whole entire life—starting tomorrow.

Later in the evening, I stand at home, alone in the kitchen after getting two restless, energetic, fighting children to bed. A two-hour ordeal; Alisa hits Zac; Zac kicks me. I haven't eaten and I need to rest. As if stuffing my face could comfort me, I raid the kitchen. Slices of banana. Chocolate chip cookie dough ice cream. Hershey's Sundae Syrup Double Chocolate Sauce. Spanish peanuts. Granola. I swirl it all around with a purple Tootsie Roll Pop until it melts and turns creamy. I slurp it standing at the counter, watching TV, reading a magazine.

> Yesterday is gone. Tomorrow has not yet come. We have only today. Let us begin.
>
> Mother Teresa

When I lift my head, I hate myself. Once again I have tried to fix boredom and fatigue with food. Yet again, I got restless and believed I couldn't stand it. The expression, "you make me sick" takes on huge meaning. I want to throw up.

I am learning heartfulness, paying attention right now on purpose, without judgment, without self-rejection, without dissociating. What can I do right now to accept myself? What would be one effort toward nurturing myself in difficult moments?

I fill the bathtub with warm, bubbly water with an herbal aromatherapy preparation for "stress relief." Sitting in the tub, I wash myself. I notice how bubbles rise, then break, how delicate the form of the shapes, and how numerous the colors. This is restful and is the beginning of the final ritual with which I end my days.

> I am still learning.
> Michelangelo

No matter if I have obliterated the day, I end my day as I began—consciously. I take five or ten minutes of in-the-heart rest in bed before falling asleep.

I used to collapse into bed to the constant badgering of the punishing voice, wake up the next day, hit the pavement running, and chastise myself all day.

Now, in a resting pose in bed, first I let go of my day and exhale to release any physical stress that remains. Bodily tension is in part the buildup of beliefs and patterns that repeat and repeat. These old habits are lessened the next day if we release them each night. Let the day go. It is past. Come into the new moment and start again.

Our son Zac had a favorite childhood book, *Goodnight Moon*. Nightly, as ritual we sang, "good night moon, good night kittens, good night mittens." Similarly, now I relax and release silently "rest, arms; rest, brain; rest, eyes; rest, legs; rest, jaw…" Giving myself permission to let go completely, I return my attention to the heart. As I started the day, so I end it, breathing in, breathing out, centered in the heart, emptying out, aware of opening to the heartfulness I will need tomorrow.

Antidotes to Food Frenzy

Find Your Heart (Twenty minutes)

Tonight before you go to bed, get comfy under the covers and then, one more time, rest in the heart.

Feel the heart. Feel into the body. Stop. Let the day melt.

Exhale a little longer than you inhale. On the exhale, let go of tension as if from the center of your chest. If you are still awake, do this for twenty minutes. You may fall asleep. If so, great; you have ended the day in your heart. No matter what happened today, end the day wholeheartedly, without making yourself wrong, letting go of any feelings of "I shoulda, coulda, woulda."

Simply let yourself be.

Let your heart radiate your life force through you and to those you love and beyond.

For twenty minutes, feel what heartfulness has done for you, is doing for you. Be heartful as you slip into dreams.

Know Thyself

In bed, review what has been right about your food that day. Even if it's "I ate one vegetable." You may have eaten mostly junk. Focus on what's working. What went well? I had a banana with breakfast. I had yummy lentil soup for lunch. What did you do that, in whatever small way, helps? **Write it down.**

Get Real with Food

Lots of experts say we sleep better if we stop eating a few hours before we sleep. To go to bed after digestion has finished helps deepen our sleep. Try it. See how you feel.

See if you can make a new habit of having a cup of herbal tea in the afternoon and evening to let the nervous system calm. Simply notice any changes.

> Go confidently in the direction of your dreams! Live the life you've imagined. As you simplify your life, the laws of the universe will be simpler.
>
> Henry David Thoreau

Afterword

Still Hungry After All These Years

> Even your body knows its heritage and
> its rightful need and will not be deceived.
> ...And now you ask in your heart,
> "How shall we distinguish that
> which is good in pleasure from
> that which is not good?"
> Go to your fields and your gardens.
>> —Kahlil Gibran, *The Prophet*

Through January, February and into Maine's March, my insides darken like the winter outside. I used to have a brilliant solution: soft brownies or something fudgy with chocolate chunks at least, or mini-chocolate chips dusted then melted on top, as much for their sheen—so needed through the season's drab—as their velvety flavor. Brownies would fix everything. That was the illusion anyway. Through frost, snow and ice, I craved the sweetness of long walks with neighbors in gentle spring breezes, summer at the beach with my cousins, playing outside in the sun with my grandsons. I sought big connections and great warmth and I headed straight to the kitchen to whip up a substitute: cocoa, sugar, butter, flour.

Heartbeat and breath rushed as I started the dance of baking. Adrenaline whispered: Brownies are what I need. Brownies will cheer me up.

Mind racing with "gotta-have-it, gotta-have it now," I threw the vanilla, the walnuts and gold box of baking soda on the soapstone countertop, clinked the metal measuring cups and played with the hollow in the plastic spoons. I folded dry ingredients into wet, poured the ribbon of thick mixture into a 9–inch square pan, and inhaled the silky scent of dark cocoa dissolving. Brownies, fun and exciting, pulled at me. I could taste their richness even as I peered through the glass oven door, peeking too soon, too often, and with just a teeny bit too much enthusiasm. I read "bake until it springs back to the touch," and finally my fingers trampolined off the spongy top.

My heart skipped. The aroma of steamy, freshly-baked brownies wafted through the condo: a smooth smell, like coffee only more robust. My stomach rumbled as the chewy confection served up a banquet for the senses and lifted me out of whatever ailed me.

For a short while.

I sampled and the ruse began. The arm and hand rhythms, the gooey scent, the licks of batter fooled me for an hour or so. But when I really paid attention, I saw that this blended brew played tricks on me. For those first few sniffs and bites—ahhhhhh—chewy chocolate made me giddy and wide-grinned. Then—after I scoffed down two, three, or four more, knife-straightened the edges, sliced squares onto a plate and devoured the morsels that fell—came a drumbeat headache and sour stomach.

Sometimes way too late, I would wake up and wonder: What did I want this physical substance to do for me?

The melt-in-the-mouth yumminess lingered a few minutes at most, picked me up and then, because it can't last, let me down. Was I looking for love in all the wrong places? The joy of indulgence, impermanent as it is, always vanishes. Brownies break, go stale, turn to crumbs and, for some of us, trouble. Before we expect brownies to fix inner and outer unwanted climate, would we be wise to ask, "What do I really want?"

It's true; some of us long for moments of chocolate relaxation and sweet-tooth satisfaction. It's also true, especially in the insistence of gotta-have-it, we could be hungering for literal and metaphoric spring in our hearts. Maybe it makes sense to turn to something larger than fleeting pleasure for ultimate sweetness. Maybe there is little wisdom in brownie-escape.

We might have to look up from our plates and beyond our taste buds to feed our soul's appetites.

Of course, we choose dessert often, and it fills us. At other times, it's possible we confuse human with spiritual yearnings, and leave our holy hungers starving, unfulfilled. Sometimes a brownie is just a brownie, a perfect antidote to winter doldrums. And sometimes, if we want no bitter aftertaste, we might have to look up from our plates and beyond our taste buds to feed our soul's appetites.

Opening the heart is transformative. Although there lingers struggle with the scars of a long war, since I have moved into my heart and since I eat a whole-foods plant-based diet, I don't fight with food any more. I am happy to know the difference, these days, between physical hunger and hunger for love, companionship, creativity or a good book, between the ravages of omnivorous appetite and true plant-based nourishment, between being full and being fulfilled. Although I still grapple with dragons, I more often dance with the heart, kindled by the inner Spark.

It makes sense to turn to something larger than fleeting pleasure for ultimate sweetness.

Am I, as a young toddler would say after kissing a boo-boo, "aw better?"

No, I am not all better, but I have kissed a very big boo-boo. I am better enough. I bow in gratitude and in celebration of the fact that I am indeed, "awe better."

You can be, too.

May we all be well.

Resources

We cannot solve a problem with the same mind that created it.

—Albert Einstein

Here are some resources that helped me move into a different "mind:" the mind of the heart.

Daily Inspirations for the Heart:

Barks, Coleman. *A Year with Rumi: Daily Readings.* San Francisco: HarperOne, 2006.

Easwarean, Eknath. *Words to Live By: Inspirations for Every Day.* Tomales, CA: Nilgiri Press, 1999.

Follmi, Danielle and Olivier. *Devotions: Wisdom from the Cradle of Civilization.* New York: Abrams, 2008.

Kornfield, Jack. *The Art of Forgiveness, Lovingkindness and Peace.* New York: Bantam Books, 2002.

Kuchler, Bonnie Louise, ed. *One Heart: Universal Wisdom from the World's Scriptures.* New York: Marlowe and Company, 2003.

McGregor, Jim. *The Tao of Recovery: A Quiet Path to Wellness.* Atlanta, GA: Humanics Publication, 1997.

Merrill, Nan with Barbara Taylor. *Peace Planet: Light for Our World.* Harpers Ferry, WV: Friends of Silence, 2006.

Norris, Gunilla. *Inviting Silence: Universal Principles of Meditation.* Katonah, NY: BlueBridge, 2004.

O'Donohue, John. *To Bless the Space Between Us.* New York: Doubleday, 2008.

Heartful Living:

Armstrong, Karen. *Twelve Steps to a Compassionate Life.* New York: Alfred A Knopf, 2010.

Brach, Tara. *Radical Acceptance: Embracing Your Life with the Heart of a Buddha.* New York: Bantam Books, 2003.

Brantley, Jeffry. *Calming Your Anxious Mind: How Mindfulness and Compassion Can Free*

You From Anxiety, Fear, and Panic. Oakland, Ca: New Harbinger Publications, 2007.

Chase, Michael. *am I being kind: how asking one simple question can change your life… and your world.* New York: Hay House, 2011.

Chodron, Pema. *Awakening Loving-kindness.* Boston: Shambhala, 1991.

Chodron, Pema. *Start Where You Are: A Guide to Compassionate Living.* Boston: Shambhala, 2001.

David, Marc. *Nourishing Wisdom: A Mind-Body Approach to Nutrition and Well-Being.* New York: Three Rivers Press, 1994.

Greenspan, Miriam. *Healing Through the Dark Emotions.* Boston: Shambhala, 2003.

Nhât Hanh, Thich. *Teachings on Love.* Berkeley: Parallax Press, 1997.

Kabat-Zinn, Jon. *Wherever You Go, There You Are.* New York: Hyperion, 1994.

Kent, Keith M. *Anyway: The Paradoxical Commandments: Finding Personal Meaning in a Crazy World.* New York: Putnam, 2001.

Kornfield, Jack. *A Path with Heart: A Guide Through the Perils and Promises of Spiritual Life.* Boston: Bantam, 1993.

Kornfield, Jack. *Buddha's Little Instruction Book.* New York: Bantam, 1994.

Kornfield, Jack. *The Wise Heart: A Guide to the Universal Teachings of Buddhist Psychology.* New York: Bantam, 2008.

Kornfield, Jack and Christina Feldman, ed. *Soul Food: Stories to Nourish the Spirit and the Heart.* San Francisco: Harper, 1996.

Levine, Stephen. *Guided Meditations, Explorations and Healings.* New York: Anchor Books, 1991.

Luhrs, Janet. *The Simple Living Guide: A Sourcebook For Less Stressful, More Joyful Living.* Boston: Broadway Books, 1997.

Makransky, John. *Awakening Through Love: Unveiling Your Deepest Goodness.* Boston: Wisdom Publications, 2007.

Neff, Kristin. *Self-Compassion: Stop Beating Yourself Up and Leave Insecurity Behind.* New York: William Morrow, 2011.

Olsen, Andrea. *Body and Earth. An Experiential Guide.* Hanover and London: University Press of New England, 2002.

Ornish, Dean. *Dr. Dean Ornish's Program for Reversing Heart Disease.* New York: Random House, 1990.

Ornish, Dean. *Love and Survival: The Scientific Basis for the Healing Power of Intimacy.* New York: Harper Collins, 1998.

Ornish, Dean. *The Spectrum: A Scientifically Proven Program to Feel Better, Live Longer, Lose Weight and Gain Health.* New York: Ballantine Books, 2007.

Paulus, Trina. *Hope for the Flowers.* New York: Paulist Press, 1972.

Remen, Rachel Naomi. *Kitchen Table Wisdom: Stories that Heal.* New York: Riverhead

Books, 1996.

Remen, Rachel Naomi. *My Grandfather's Blessings: Stories of Strength, Refuge, and Belonging.* New York: Riverhead Books, 2001.

Robbins, John and Ann Mortifee. *In Search of Balance: Discovering Harmony in a Changing World.* Tiburon, CA: H J Kramer, Inc., 1991.

Santorelli, Saki. *Heal Thy Self: Lessons on Mindfulness in Medicine.* New York: Three Rivers Press, 2000.

Seid, Roberta Pollack. *Never Too Thin: Why Women are at War with Their Bodies.* New York: Prentice Hall Press, 1989.

Stahl, Bob and Steve Flowers. *Living with Your Heart Wide Open: How Mindfulness and Compassion Can Free You from Unworthiness, Inadequacy and Shame.* Oakland, CA: New Harbinger Publications, 2011.

Straub, Gail. *The Rhythm of Compassion: Caring for Self, Connecting with Society.* West Hurley, NY: Empowerment Institute, 2008.

Taylor, Shelley E. *The Tending Instinct: How Nurturing is Essential to Who We Are and How We Live.* New York: Henry Holt & Co., 2002.

Welwood, John, ed. *Awakening the Heart: East/West Approaches to Psychotherapy and the Healing Relationship.* Boulder, CO: Shambhala, 1983.

Whyte, David. *The Heart Aroused: Poetry and the Preservation of Soul in Corporate America.* New York: Currency Doubleday, 1994.

Internet Resources for Heartful Living

Tara Brach's website: tarabrach.com

The Center for Mindfulness www.umassmed.edu/cfm/

The Compassionate Mind Foundation: comapssionatemind.co.uk

The Dalai Lama's website: dalailama.com

The Food Revolution: www.foodrevolution.org

The ToDo Institute: http://todoinstitute.org/

Kritin Neff's self-compassion website: www.self-compassion.org

www.yourheartwideopen.com

www.mindfulnessprograms.com/mindful-healing-series.html.

www.mindfullivingprograms.com

Journaling and Writing

Cameron, Julia. *The Writing Diet: Write Yourself Right-Size.* New York: Tarcher, 2007.

Capacchione, Lucia, Elizabeth Johnson and James Strohecker. *Lighten Up Your Body, Lighten Up Your Life: Beyond Diet & Exercise.* North Hollywood, CA; Newcastle Publishing, 1990.

DeSalvo, Louise. *Writing as a Way of Healing: How Telling Our Stories Transforms Our Lives.* Boston: Beacon Press, 2000.

Herring, Laraine. *Writing Begins with the Breath: Embodying Your Authentic Voice.* Boston: Shambhala, 2007.

Newman, Leslea. *Write From the Heart: Inspiration and Exercises for Women Who Want to Write.* Berkeley, CA: Ten Speed Press, 2003.

Ueland, Brenda. *If You Want to Write: A Book About Art, Independence and Spirit.* Saint Paul, MN: Graywolf Press, 1987.

Heartful Eating

Albers, Susan. *Eat, Drink and Be Mindful: How to End Your Struggle with Mindless Eating and Start Savoring Food with Intention and Joy.* Oakland, CA: New Harbinger, 2008.

Bays, Jan Chozen. *Mindful Eating: A Guide to Rediscovering a Healthy and Joyful Relationship with Food.* Boston: Shambhala, 2009.

Fain, Jean. *The Self-Compassion Diet: A Step-by-Step Program to Lose Weight with Loving-Kindness.* Boulder, CO: Sounds True, 2010.

Hanh, Thich Nhat, and Cheung, Lilian. *Savor: Mindful Eating, Mindful Life.* New York: Harper One, 2011.

Kano, Susan. *Making Peace with Food.* New York: William Morrow Paperbacks, 1989.

Kessler, David. *The End of Overeating: Taking Control the Insatiable American Appetite.* New York: Rodale, 2009.

Wansink, Brian. *Mindless Eating: Why We Eat More than We Think.* New York: Bantam Books, 2006.

Yuen, Carmen. *The Cosmos in a Carrot: A Zen Guide to Eating Well.* Berkeley, CA: Parallax Press, 2006.

Internet Resources for Heartful Eating

Susan Alber's Eat, Drink, and Be Mindful: eatingmindfully.org
The Center for Mindful Eating: tcme.org
The Conscious Café: theconsciouscafe.org

Resources

Heartful Movement:

Devi, Nischala Joy. *The Healing Path of Yoga: Alleviate Stress, Open Your Heart and Enrich Your Life.* New York: Three Rivers Press, 2000.

Dreyer, Canny and Katherine. *Chi Walking: Fitness Walking for Lifelong Health.* New York: Simon & Schuster, 2006.

Farhi, Donna. *Yoga Mind, Body and Spirit: A Return to Wholeness.* New York: Henry Holt and Company, 2000.

Galway, W. Tim. *Inner Game of Golf.* New York: Random House, 1998.

Galway, W. Tim. *Inner Game of Tennis.* New York: Random House, 1997.

Gershon, David. *Soft Running: The Next Step.* New York: Amity House, 1985.

Heidrich, Ruth E. *Senior Fitness: The Diet and Exercise Program for Maximum Health and Longevity.* New York: Lantern Books, 2005.

Kortge, Carolyn Scott. *Healing Walks for Hard Times: Quiet Your Mind, Strengthen Your Body, and Get Your Life Back.* Boston: Trumpeter, 2010.

Nhât Hanh, Thích and Wietske Vreizen. *Mindful Movement.* Berkeley, CA: Parallax Press, 2008.

Heartful Nutrition

(*= includes recipes)

Barnard, Neal. *Breaking the Food Seduction: The Hidden Reasons Behind Food Cravings and 7 Steps to End Them Naturally.* New York: St. Martin's Press, 2003.*

Barnard, Neal. *Eat Right, Live Longer: Using the Natural Power of Foods to Age-Proof Your Body.* New York: Three Rivers Press, 1995.

Barnard, Neal. *Turn Off Your Fat Genes.* New York: Harmony Books, 2001.

Barnard, Neal. *21-Day Weight Loss Kickstart: Boost Metabolism, Lower Cholesterol, and Dramatically Improve Your Health.* New York: Hachette Book Group, 2011. *

Brazier, Brendan. *The Thrive Diet: The Whole Foods Way to Losing Weight, Reducing Stress, and Staying Healthy for Life.* Philadelphia, PA: Da Capo Lifelong, 2007. *

Brazier, Brendan. *Thrive Fitness: The Vegan-Based Training Program for Maximum Strength, Health and Fitness.* Philadelphia, PA: Da Capo Lifelong, 2009. *

Campbell, T. Colin and Thomas Campbell. *The China Study: Startling Implications for Diet, Weight Loss, and Long-Term Health.* Dallas, TX: BenBella Books, 2006.

Chef AJ and Glen Merzer. *Unprocessed: How to Achieve Vibrant Health and Your Ideal Weight.* USA: CreateSpace, 2011.*

Esselstyn, Caldwell. *Prevent and Reverse Heart Disease: The Revolutionary, Scientifically Proven, Nutrition-Based Cure.* New York: Avery, 2007. *

Resources

Esselstyn, Rip. *The Engine 2 Diet: The Texas Firefighter's 28-day Save-Your-Life Plan that Lowers Cholesterol and Burns Away the Pounds.* New York: Wellness Central, 2009. *

Fuhrman, Joel. *Eat For Health: Lose Weight, Keep It Off, Look Younger, Live Longer.* Flemington, NJ; Gift of Health Press, 2008. *

Fuhrman, Joel. *Eat To Live: The Revolutionary Formula for Fast and Sustained Weight Loss.* Boston: Little Brown and Company, 2003.*

Fuhrman, Joel. *Nutritarian Handbook and Andi Food Scoring Guide.* USA: Nutritional Excellence, LLC, 2010.

Havala, Suzanne. *The Natural Kitchen: Your Guide to the Sustainable Food Revolution.* Berkeley, CA: Process, 2010.

Hever, Julieanna. *The Complete Idiot's Guide to Plant-Based Nutrition.* New York: Penguin Group, 2011.*

Goldhamer, Alan. *The Health Promoting Cookbook: Simple, Guilt-Free, Vegetarian Recipes.* Summertown, TN: Book Publishing Company, 1997. *

Lanou, Amy Joy and Michael Castleman. *Building Bone Vitality: A Revolutionary Diet Plan to Prevent Bone Loss and Reverse Osteoporosis.* New York: McGraw Hill, 2009. *

Lisle, Douglas and Alan Goldhamer. *The Pleasure Trap.* Summertown, TN: Healthy Living Publications, 2003.

Moran, Victoria. *Love-Powered Diet: Eating for Freedom, Health, and Joy.* Herndon, VA: Lantern Books, 2009.

Nearing, Helen. *Simple Food for the Good Life: An Alternative Cookbook.* New York: Delacorte Press, 1980. *

Nixon, Lindsay S. *The Happy Herbivore Cookbook: Over 175 Delicious Fat-Free and Low-Fat Vegan Recipes.* Dallas, TX: BenBella Books, 2011.*

Pollan, Michael. *Food Rules: An Eater's Manual.* New York: Penguin, 2009.

Popper, Pam. *Dr. Pam Popper's Guide to Family Health and Wellness.* Elk Grove Village, IL: P.B. Industries, 2006.

Pulde, Alona, and Matthew Lederman. *Keep It Simple, Keep It Whole: Your Guide to Optimum Health.* Los Angeles, CA: Exsalus Health and Wellness Center, 2010. *

Raymond, Jennifer. *The Peaceful Palate.* Calistoga, CA: Heart and Soul Publication, 1992.*

Raymond, Jennifer. *Fat-Free and Easy: Great Meals in Minutes.* Calistoga, CA: Heart and Soul Publications, 1995. *

Silverstone, Alicia. *The Kind Diet: A Simple Guide to Feeling Great, Losing Weight, and Saving the Planet.* New York: Rodale, 2009.*

Stephens, Arran and Eliot Jay Rosen. *The Compassionate Diet: How What You Eat Can Change Your Life and Save the Planet.* New York: Rodale, 2011.

Stone, Gene, ed. *Forks Over Knives.* New York: The Experiment, 2011*

Resources

Internet Resources for Heartful Nutrition

www.brendadavisrd.com
www.ChefAJsHealthyKitchen.com
www.ChowDownMovie.com
www.drfuhrman.com
www.exalus.com
www.happycow.net
www.happyherbivore.net
www.heartattackproof.com
www.todoinstitute.org
www.pcrm.org
www.plantbaseddiet.com
www.tcolincampbell.org
www.theengine2diet.com
www.wellnessforum.com
www.plantbaseddietician.com

Films on Heartful Nutrition:

Chow Down Movie
Fat, Sick and Nearly Dead
Food, Inc.
Forks over Knives
Planeat
Supersize
To your Health: A Journey into the Plant-Based World by Julieanna Hever

Heartful Caring for Animals and the Environment:

Brazier, Brendan. *Thrive Foods: 200 Plant-Based Recipes for Peak Health*. Philadelphia, PA: Da Capo Lifelong, 2011.*

Coats, C. David. *Old MacDonald's Factory Farm*. New York: Continuum Publishing, 1989.

Foer, Jonathan Saffran. *Eating Animals*. New York: Little, Brown and Company, 2009.

Lappe, Frances Moore and Anna Lappé. *Hope's Edge: The Next Diet for a Small Planet*. New York: Tarcher/Putnam, 2003.

Lyman, Howard and Glen Merzer. *Mad Cowboy*. New York: Simon & Schuster, 1998.

Lyman, Howard, Glen Merzer and Joanna Samorow-Merzer. *No More Bull!* New York: Scriber, 2005.

Masson, Jeffrey Moussaieff and McCarthy, Susan. *When Elephants Weep: The Emotional Lives of Animals.* New York: Delacorte, 1995.

Rifkin, Jeremy. *Beyond Beef: The Rise and Fall of the Cattle Culture.* New York: Dutton, 1992.

Robbins, John. *Diet for a New America.* Tiburon, CA: H.J. Kramer, 1998.

Robbins, John. *The Food Revolution: How Your Diet Can Help Save Your Life and Our World.* Berkeley, CA: Conari Press, 2001.

Robbins, John and Gia Patton. *May All Be Fed: A Diet for A New World.* William Morrow and Company, 1992.

Stepaniak, Joanne. *Compassionate Living for Healing, Wholeness and Harmony.* New York: McGraw-Hill, 2001.

Memoirs of Heartless Eating and Recovery

De Rossi, Portia. *Unbearable Lightness: A Story of Loss and Gain.* New York: Atria Book, 2010.

Knapp, Caroline. *Appetites: Why Women Want.* New York: Counterpoint, 2003.

Seles, Monica. *Getting a Grip: On My Body, My Mind, My Self.* New York: Avery, 2009.

Schaefer, Jenni with Thom Rutledge. *Life Without Ed: How One Woman Declared Independence from Her Eating Disorder and How You Can Too.* New York: McGraw Hill, 2003.

The Brain, Biochemistry and Food Frenzy

Barnard, Neal. *Breaking the Food Seduction.* New York: St. Martin's Press, 2003. *

Fuhrman, Joel. *Eat For Health: Lose Weight; Keep it Off; Look Younger: Live Longer.* Flemington, NJ: Gift of Health Press, 2008. *

Lisle, Douglas and Alan Goldhamer. *The Pleasure Trap.* Summertown, TN: Healthy Living Publications, 2003.

About the Author

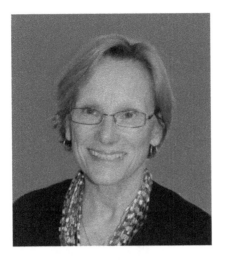

Susan Lebel Young MSED, MSC, author of *Lessons From A Golfer: A Daughter's Story of Opening the Heart, Grandkids as Gurus: Lessons for Grownups,* is a perfect guide on your journey toward heartfulness in your food and life. Young is a self-professed junk food junkie who has maintained a fifty pound weight loss and a change of food-frenzy mentality for thirty years using these food fix antidotes. She has Masters degrees in both Education and Counseling. She has studied and taught mindfulness in Maine, South Carolina and at the Center for Mindfulness at the University of Massachusetts Medical School. Young has helped clients in her private psychotherapy practice since 1995 and taught yoga since 2000. She has led mindfulness workshops, taught mindful eating, and taught courses that she developed in mind-body approaches to counseling and spirituality in the counseling process to Master's level counseling students. Young studied plant-based nutrition with *The China Study* author T. Colin Campbell's e-Cornell courses. She writes a column "Life Unwound" in the weekly *Forecaster.*

Young is a very proud grandmother, mother of two adult children, and lives with her husband Jon in Falmouth, Maine.

Susan is available to workshops and speaking engagements. For more information go to:

www.SusanLebelYoung.com

CPSIA information can be obtained
at www.ICGtesting.com
Printed in the USA
FSHW021044080521
81249FS

9 781934 949528